The AIDS Generation:

Stories of Survival and Resilience

PERRY N. HALKITIS

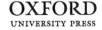
OXFORD
UNIVERSITY PRESS

OXFORD
UNIVERSITY PRESS

Oxford University Press is a department of the University of Oxford.
It furthers the University's objective of excellence in research, scholarship,
and education by publishing worldwide.

Oxford   New York
Auckland   Cape Town   Dar es Salaam   Hong Kong   Karachi
Kuala Lumpur   Madrid   Melbourne   Mexico City   Nairobi
New Delhi   Shanghai   Taipei   Toronto

With offices in
Argentina   Austria   Brazil   Chile   Czech Republic   France   Greece
Guatemala   Hungary   Italy   Japan   Poland   Portugal   Singapore
South Korea   Switzerland   Thailand   Turkey   Ukraine   Vietnam

Published in the United States of America by
Oxford University Press
198 Madison Avenue, New York, NY 10016

Library of Congress Cataloging in Publication Data
Halkitis, Perry N., author.
The AIDS generation : stories of survival and resilience / Perry N. Halkitis.
   p. ; cm.
Includes bibliographical references and index.
ISBN 978–0–19–994497–2 (alk. paper)
I. Title.
[DNLM: 1. Acquired Immunodeficiency Syndrome—United States—Personal
Narratives.   2. Epidemics—history—United States—Personal Narratives.   3. HIV
Long-Term Survivors—United States—Personal Narratives.   4. History, 20th Century—
United States—Personal Narratives.   5. History, 21st Century—United States—Personal
Narratives.   6. Homosexuality, Male—psychology—United States—Personal Narratives.
WC 503]
RA643.8
614.5′99392—dc23
2013023760

9 8 7 6 5 4 3 2
Printed in the United States of America
on acid-free paper

Dedication
For my two Roberts

CONTENTS

Shortly after 10 a.m. on December 18, 2012, my old friend Spencer Cox drew his last breath. He was 44.

He hadn't looked very healthy when I saw him 7 weeks earlier. There was an unusual greenish tint in his skin and he appeared to have lost weight. His clothing—oversized jeans and an old blue plaid shirt with buttons missing—billowed over his crooked frame, which once had been so admirable. This poor impression was further enhanced by the pirate's patch he wore over his now nonfunctioning left eye, and the smell of too many cigarettes.

He spoke of feeling run down, an understatement it turns out. What killed him was old-fashioned AIDS: no CD4 cells, a viral load in the millions, and fluids filling his lungs—this, despite the fact that he'd lived over half his life in HIV care and personally knew the world's top infectious disease doctors and researchers. In fact, as a veteran AIDS activist he helped those researchers study and then roll out protease inhibitors, the game-changing drugs that hit the market in 1996 and finally slowed the dying. But when friends gathered at his apartment to pack up his belongings—that funereal routine from the '80s and '90s—they found bottles of unopened medicine. Inexplicably, Spencer had gone off the pills.

Why had he done that? There was much hand-wringing among family and friends, but not among people who saw what Spencer saw, who had been through what so many of us had—events that Perry Halkitis and the men whose voices he amplifies in this volume describe in explicit detail. We are survivors of the plague years in America from 1981 to 1996, when death came cold and often, a world-gone-mad era when hospitals would deny us care, churches refused us succor, and our own beloved families angrily left us for dead. We carry deep wounds from this time. The death memories haunt us. In the last year of the plague alone, nearly as many young Americans died of AIDS as perished in the Vietnam War.

Soldiers returning from Indochina were said to have war trauma. And us? Ours is a condition we know so little about. Some are calling it AIDS survivors syndrome, with its unfortunate acronym. Halkitis gives it affirmation for the first time here. He writes: "In truth, the gay men of my generation, the AIDS Generation—all of us, HIV-positive or negative, across every race, ethnicity, and culture, from every part of our country, from stockbroker to dancer to salesman—were robbed of a life filled with youthful frivolity, with endless optimism and hope. And as middle-aged men, we are as a group traumatized and fatigued from 30 years of war."

That was Spencer. He had been an actor before being diagnosed at 19. He handled the news with Spencerian aplomb. He wrote: "So my counselor says, 'I won't keep you in suspense—you're positive.' And then, while I'm calculating my life expectancy, she says, 'But the good news is, your syphilis test came back negative.' She was surprised that I laughed. When you test positive, everyone seems to expect you to turn into Sylvia Plath."

Despite having no formal training, for the next decade he threw himself into the scientific work that today allows 8 million people to control their HIV. But the plague's end was as disorienting as it was a relief. It threw Spencer out of the only adult life he had ever known, a high-wire act as amplified and brilliant as anybody in wartime has experienced. In surviving, we accomplished extraordinary feats. Yet we delivered ourselves into a depleted and lonely world.

Too often, our experiences were no longer esteemed. Spencer, whose advice was sought by Nobel Laureates, was now sidelined—not a real scientist and a decade away from the promising acting career he had put on hold, he was just a man who took pills now. His jobs grew stale and friends drifted away. What a terrible irony, to have battled for an ordinary life, then to be unable to enjoy one.

He turned to methamphetamines at one point—a lot of the survivors did. That got him off his AIDS meds the first time, sent him to the hospital with pneumonia and retinitis, and robbed him of that left eye. Thereafter, a profound depression and recurring health issues kept him reliant upon social services. He didn't talk about this with friends. But he was an avid poster on Gawker, where a few weeks before the end he used a nom de plume (revealed after his death) to pull back the curtain on his life:

> Some days, I'm fine, and get around with no problem. Other days, I'm curled in fetal position in bed the whole day (and more often, several days), racked with pain the whole time. Some days I'm on the subway getting the stink-eye from some old or pregnant lady who clearly wants my seat, and can't tell just by looking at me that I'm sitting because I'm on my way home from a doctor's appointment, and if I stand for one more minute, I'm going to fall on the ground.

After he died, some who had worked with him cursed Spencer for being careless with his life. Others have wondered if Spencer's death was a suicide—had he indeed turned into Sylvia Plath? But these guesses miss the point. What killed Spencer? The plague killed Spencer—the hideous experience of those long years did him in. As was said about the great Holocaust writer Primo Levi, after he plunged to his death as a sad old man, Spencer Cox never left the camps. Maybe none of us have.

In the following pages you will find the voices of 15 survivors from this medieval time not so long ago—including Halkitis. And through their voices you will begin to be able to see the faces of the countless young men they held at the end. As you're reading, close your eyes from time to time and let the plague come back in all its complexity and contradiction: emaciated bodies and an inability anymore to cry, and an amazing sense of purpose, community, and love—for our community, and for ourselves. It is possible to miss that time, as awful as that seems, and not just because there are so many people we miss from then. A friend once said to me, "We had so much fun when everybody was dying," by which he meant, "We comported ourselves admirably and with great purpose, alongside a community of brave men and women, whom we came to love."

Listen closely to the words of Ralph, when you find them. He speaks for all AIDS survivors. "Our experiences write our history," he will tell you. "Without these experiences I wouldn't have been or become who I am now. And so although I didn't really *enjoy* it, I *appreciate* it."

David France is a longtime AIDS journalist, author, and filmmaker. His book "Our Fathers" was a national best seller and his Oscar-nominated documentary "How to Survive a Plague" won numerous awards.

*T*he *AIDS Generation* has resided in some shape and form in my mind for close to a decade. Although I bring to this volume the approaches and stances of a scientist who has been studying the lives of gay men and the impact of HIV/AIDS for the last two decades, I also bring to this work my own life experiences as a gay man who came of age as the AIDS epidemic emerged—as a member of the AIDS Generation. This work touches many facets of my existence. It is surely a scientific work, but also an act of love and an affirmation of life.

The approach I have taken to writing this book is directed by two goals: (1) to add to the current academic knowledge and (2) to appeal to a larger audience who resides beyond the walls of academia. Mostly, I sought to demonstrate the strength, courage, and resilience of my generation of gay men and to document our ability to survive a plague. It is my hope that this work will enhance the discourse about HIV and our efforts to defeat this epidemic. However, this book will have even greater impact if it empowers gay men, especially a new generation of gay men, both locally and globally to be activists for their rights and their health. Finally, I also wrote this book lest the world forget the pain and suffering through which my generation of gay men lived.

I am grateful to the men of the AIDS Generation who have shared their life stories with me and have allowed me to share them with you throughout this volume. I have selected these 15 men because of their diverse life experiences and existences. In telling their stories, my goal was to show that there is more than one story of AIDS, that there are many interesting and complex stories, unified only by a set of common conditions. These beautiful, intelligent, and powerful men have enriched my life and helped me better understand my own place in the world. I am confident that their stories will serve as an inspiration to anyone who reads this book. From these life histories, we all can glean important life lessons about survival, resilience, and dignity. To these amazing and inspirational men, this book is you!

The AIDS Generation takes you on a peripatetic journey, interweaving the stories of these men with my own experiences as a gay man who came of age in the 1980s and witnessed the emergence and evolution of HIV/ AIDS, the robust scientific literature on the disease, and the media and other artistic reactions to the epidemic. I have structured the book along six chapters. In the first chapter, we consider socio-historical realities of HIV/AIDS in the lives of gay men. In Chapter 2, I provide an overview of the research process that was enacted to gather the data and I offer a description of the 15 men whose stories constitute the center of this book. In Chapters 3 and 4, I examine how the men came to know their lives as HIV-positive, the devastation and loss in their lives, and their strategies for survival. The experience of aging is then considered in Chapter 5, and in Chapter 6, I conclude by demonstrating how the life experiences of the men of the AIDS Generation inform a model of resilience, although the resilience and power of these men is evident throughout the course of the volume.

No man walks through life alone. This idea is exemplified in the stories of the men of the AIDS Generation, and it is highly relevant to the writing of this book. As always, I am indebted to my research team at the Center for Health, Identity, Behavior, and Prevention Studies (CHIBPS) at New York University (NYU) for their dedication to the fight against AIDS and the work that they undertake on daily basis—work that is more than an intellectual exercise and a means toward a degree for them. Other scientists may struggle with the translation of their work and the meaning it has to real people in real lives, but we live it. Particular thanks to my students Sandy Kupprat, Francesca Bates, Jessica Eddy, and Molly Kingdon, and to my post-doc Rafael Perez Figueroa for helping me enact the research program that is the basis of this book and for their ongoing enthusiasm while I was writing this volume, as well as to Alvaro Moreira, who helped me bring this project to a close. Also, my sincere appreciation to my research partner Farzana Kapadia for her collaborative spirit and for keeping the trains running at CHIBPS while I took the time to write the book.

Words of gratitude are insufficient for my colleague and friend Nancy Hall. She has been my muse, has walked by my side as this project emerged, and was a source of strength, wisdom, and insight, especially as I struggled with the very challenging emotions that were evoked in the writing process. As a woman who came of age in the 1980s in New York City, her life too was affected by the devastation of AIDS. She too is part of the AIDS Generation.

Finally, to NYU's Senior Vice President for Health Bob Berne, many thanks for the support he provided me to undertake this research and for his unwavering belief in me as a significant voice in the public health discourse.

I have dedicated *The AIDS Generation* to my two Roberts—Robert Massa and Bobby Halkitis—the bookends of my life. Like so many gay men, Robert lost his battle to AIDS in 1994. My work is because of him. My husband Bobby has brought the life back into my life, which freed me from the past and has allowed me to write this book for you.

CHAPTER 1 | 30 Years and Counting
The Story of AIDS in the Gay Community

I KNOW NO ADULT life without AIDS. Like the long-term survivors you will come to know in the pages that follow, all of the gay men of my generation, infected or not, are long-term survivors of this disease. We were all affected by AIDS as we emerged into our adult lives, trying to avoid the end product of this pathogen—a termination to our existences in the prime of our lives. Yet like a subset of these men who became infected early in the epidemic and remain vibrant and healthy 30 years later, all of us—my generation—have survived this plague, battle scarred but resilient and stronger individually and as a community. It has been said that Americans who served in World War II are the greatest generation. I say that my generation, the generation of gay men who came into their own in the 1970s and 1980s and were decimated by AIDS, are, instead, the bravest generation. I know it because I lived it.

The story of AIDS is not a simple one. In recent years it has been drilled into our heads that HIV/AIDS is a disease that affects all Americans. Epidemiological trends certainly suggest that the virus has no boundaries and that countless others who are not gay men have become infected (Centers for Disease Control and Prevention [CDC], 2013a). Despite the prevalence of HIV/AIDS in all segments of the population, the epidemic in the United States has always been and still is, and likely will continue to be, primarily a gay disease. Many, including activist Gabrielle Rotello (1997), have provided multifaceted explanations for why AIDS happened to gay men, and there is sufficient reason to believe that there are myriad biological, medical, behavioral, political, sexual, and social factors at play.

But my point here is not *why* AIDS happened to us, but rather that AIDS did happen to us—a disease that now has affected up to three generations of gay men.

As of 2011, it is estimated that 1.1 million people are living with HIV infection in the United States, and close to 650,000 have died to date, resulting in close to 2 million cases since the onset of the epidemic (CDC, 2013a). In the 30 years since the CDC starting tracking, over 50% of those who have died are gay men (albeit the CDC labels us as "men who have sex with men" rather than "gay," an issue I will later address); more than 50% of those currently infected and living with the disease are gay men; and over 50% of new infections detected in any given year are in gay men, mostly young gay men of color. This 50% far exceeds the 2% to 5% of the population that recent surveillance indicates we constitute (Chandra, Mosher, Copen, & Sionean, 2011). As I write this book, 550,000 cases have been noted among gay men, associated with a quarter-million AIDS-related deaths (CDC, 2013a).

At the onset of the epidemic and for a short period thereafter, the strange disease that was afflicting what should have been perfectly healthy young gay men was named GRID (gay-related immune deficiency), since at the time only gay men seemed to be infected and affected (Oswald, Theodossi, Gazzard, Byrom, & Fisher-Hoch, 1982). Within the same period, the disease also was known as the more inclusive CRID (community-related immune deficiency) and as the more inflammatory "gay cancer." Given the prevalence of the affliction among gay men, it was postulated that it was our lifestyles—multiple sexual partners and drug use—that damaged our immune systems, making us susceptible to the disease. Immune overload (Goedert et al., 1982) and use of butyl and amyl nitrates (Gottlieb et al., 1981) were indicated as potential reasons for the epidemic. Although our sexual lives and use of poppers are not the direct causes of the disease, an assumption that was refuted with the identification of the HIV-1 virus in 1985 by scientists in both France and the United States (Connor & Kingman, 1988), these two factors are often implicated in the acquisition of the disease, simply not in a causal manner. In the epidemiological paradigm known as the sufficient-components model (Aschengrau & Seage, 2008), multiple sex partners and illicit drug use are potential cofactors of the disease or components of the cause, but HIV is the necessary cause. Without the presence of HIV infection there is no disease, or rather use of poppers alone or multiple sex partners alone will not cause HIV infection in the absence of the viral transmission.

At that time, attention to AIDS was rather limited and only appeared briefly in the major media outlets. The summer before college and immediately preceding my life as a gay man, I read Lawrence Altman's very brief article in *The New York Times*, "Rare Cancer Seen in 41 Homosexuals" (Altman, 1981). At the end of my first year of college and my first sexual encounters with men, I read with concern, "New Homosexual Disorder Worries Health Officials" (Altman, 1982a). Thirty years later GRID/CRID/gay cancer is now known as HIV/AIDS, and although gay lifestyle per se is not believed to be the direct cause of the disease, HIV/AIDS is for the most part a gay epidemic in the United States and the industrialized world. The disease is indicative of a health disparity in gay men (Halkitis, Wolitksi, & Millett, 2013).

It is because this plague first affected gay men (and continues to bombard us) that Ronald Reagan ignored it. It is one of the reasons George W. Bush instead turned his attention to the African AIDS epidemic. This is also likely the reason that for the first 30 years of the epidemic our country did not have a national AIDS policy (White House Office of National AIDS Policy, 2010). The Obama administration finally openly acknowledged the havoc AIDS had created in the United States, and for gay men—for my generation, the Stonewall generation that preceded us, and now a new generation of millennials, who were born into a world where AIDS is a global pandemic and a reality of their lives.

Because HIV/AIDS is primarily a gay disease in the United States and because early understandings associated the disease with our lifestyle, it also is the reason that much of heterosexual America turned their backs on us and pointed their collective finger at our lifestyle. Describing the condition at the time, Randy Shilts wrote, in his seminal work *And the Band Played On* (1987, p. 352),

> The Alert Citizens of Texas inflamed local fears with their brochure "The Gay Plague," which provided detailed descriptions of bathhouses, rimming, and golden showers. A nationally distributed Moral Majority Report also explored every unsavory aspect of gay life in gory full-color detail. And Rev. Jerry Falwell now told concerned Americans that they could fight the spread of AIDS by giving money to him.

Moreover, because of these circumstances at the onset of the AIDS epidemic, the gay rights movement, having gained so much momentum in the 1970s, came to a screeching halt. Quite simply, this epidemic derailed all of our lives physically, emotionally, socially, and politically.

Describing reactions to cancer, Susan Sontag writes (1977) that many individuals afflicted with this disease have found themselves shunned by relatives and friends and are objects of the practices of decontamination, as if their disease was infectious. One need only keep this in mind in imagining the reactions to those afflicted with an actual infectious disease, HIV/AIDS, or recall the panicked reactions of the world when it was revealed that Greg Louganis was HIV-positive at the time of the 1988 Olympics when he hit his head on the diving board and bled in the pool. Sadly for this great sports hero, this final victory of an illustrious career was filled with thoughts of doubt and shame created by our society: "What would the people cheering for me think if they knew I was gay and HIV-positive? Would they still cheer? And lurking in the back of my mind was the fear that I might have infected someone with HIV following my accident" (Louganis & Marcus, 1995, p. 213). At this point of the epidemic, with homophobia and AIDSphobia very present in our lives, as many of us were dying, and as much of society simply viewed us as vessels of a deadly disease, we had no choice but to attend to our individual and collective health. We had to attend to helping those overcome by the disease, combating the vitriol hurled upon us because of AIDS, in effect making any work toward progressing our civil rights as gay men an impossibility.

Much progress had been made since the Stonewall Riots of 1969, which marks the beginning of the gay rights era (Duberman, 1994). Within a decade, "gay" had become a mainstream term, albeit one that continued to be associated with a character disorder, and "homosexual" was the term favored by most media outlets and most Americans up until recently. Although both the American Psychiatric Association and the American Psychological Association had removed homosexuality as an illness from its list of mental disorders in the early 1970s (Bayer, 1987), a gay lifestyle was still taboo. As gay men flocked to their meccas in New York City and San Francisco, our presence was beginning to be felt—on television, in film, and in politics. Think of Billy Crystal's character Jodie Dallas on *Soap* (a stereotypical character who eventually becomes straight), and Steven Carrington, who experiences the wrath of his homophobic father on the first season of *Dynasty*. Recall the major motion pictures of the time that were gay themed—*Making Love* and *Cruising*—albeit not flattering portrayals of gay men, as Vito Russo indicates in *The Celluloid Closet* (1987); still, our presence was being noted. But mostly think of the incredible Harvey Milk and the possibilities that his presence and voice created for us!

Many of my generation entered our teens and young adulthood in this historical period of the 1970s and 1980s with a sense of confidence and zeal due to the efforts of our predecessors, the Stonewall generation—who spent years hiding their identity—demanding their rights and easing the path for us. We had also the energy of the civil rights and women's rights movements to support us. This is not to say that we came into our own with ease and without fear. Many of us still remained in our closet throughout our high school years for fear of being found out to be a faggot. Still, the promise for sexual freedom and sexual expression existed within our grasp. Little were we to know that we would become the AIDS Generation, and that within a decade this deadly disease would destroy our physical, emotional, and social lives. I know this because I am part of the AIDS Generation (Halkitis, 2011).

The Story of AIDS in Gay Men

The story of AIDS and gay men takes many forms. For me it is primarily the story of Robert Massa (1995), my partner for 6 years, an accomplished writer and journalist who turned his attention from the world of theater to the world of AIDS after he was diagnosed. It is the story of his struggle to remain healthy, by ingesting a formulation of lipid extracted from egg yolks (AL721), a holistic treatment many used in the absence of any effective antiviral treatments. On road trips Robert would place his "treatment," which was sold in soy sauce plastic packaging and looked like yellow mustard, in a cooler to keep it from spoiling. He also wrote in his columns for *The village voice* about these therapies that he administered to his weakening body to stay alive—egg yolks and Chinese cucumbers. He was livid about the misinterpretation of the effectiveness of the highly caustic first HIV antiviral treatment AZT by *The New York Times* (Massa, 1990). Robert died in 1994, 2 years before highly effective therapies might have saved his life.

It is also the story of Jim, a man double my age when we met while I was first coming out, who introduced me to the gay scene, and who was one of the earliest victims of the epidemic. He suffered in silence as his immune system failed, only to develop lymphoma, which ravaged his body before he died in 1986. No one recorded this as an AIDS death, but it was just that. It was all very quiet and concealed. I remember the day he died. It was the day after the Challenger space crew carrying schoolteacher Christa McAuliffe exploded. Americans were shattered by this tragedy.

We as gay men were suffering our own disaster silently and with much more circumscribed outcries of love and support.

It is the story of Tony, my friend who left his working-class roots of New Jersey to establish himself as a well-regarded interior designer in New York City. He was my Macy's shopping buddy. When cryptosporidiosis, a parasitic infection, overtook his digestive system in 1993, his kind Italian American mother sat at his side until the pain was gone. At his wake, a group of us, his gay family, made our way to the suburbs of New Jersey to witness a mourning and remembrance that paid no honor to his "real" life. His partner at the time, Frank, who would die a few years later, was designated to the seating at the rear of the hall, not up front with the family. (The story of Frank might now seem cliché, but it only became so because it happened so often to so many gay men throughout the epidemic.)

And it is the stories of Rick and Cameron, one a graphic designer from the foothills of the Blue Ridge Mountains of North Carolina, the other a chef from the shores of Lake Superior in Canada. Both managed to survive past 1996, marked by many as the turning point in our war against AIDS, but their bodies were already too destroyed to make effective use of the new treatments. Yes, people continue to die from complications of AIDS.

These indeed are the stories of AIDS in my life; they are the ones of loss and remembrance. They are the stories that have in many ways shaped the path of my research, and these are the stories that have led me to the writing of this book. You see, neither Robert, nor Jim, nor Tony, nor Rick, nor Cameron made it to their 50th birthdays. For that matter, Robert, Tony, and Jim didn't even make it to 40.

It is also the story of artist and activist Michael Callen. In 1990, Callen's provocative book *Surviving AIDS* was published. In that seminal work, Callen explored the stories of long-term survivors, men who like himself had controlled the disease for 8 years at the time his book was published, despite the fact that only 20% of those diagnosed before January 1, 1985, were still alive. In *Surviving AIDS*, Callen grapples with a methodology to enumerate long-term survivors, only to conclude that just 1 in 10 men diagnosed early in the epidemic, in the 1980s, were fortunate enough to be long-term survivors. For these men, the lack of effective detection of the disease meant that many were identified as infected only long after they had developed AIDS, only when symptoms emerged, and when the health care provided could only manage the opportunistic infections but not control the underlying infection with HIV. Callen attributed his survival, which at the time was quite remarkable, to "Luck, Classic Coke, and the Love of a good man." Michael died in 1993, at age 38.

Today, of course, the AIDS epidemic in the United States has radically shifted due to medical advances—the detection of HIV-1 followed by the development of the HIV antibody test in the mid-1980s and ultimately the discovery of highly effective therapies a decade later. HIV antibody tests can yield results within 20 minutes through oral fluids, and a home testing kit has been developed. Antivirals exist in multitudes and across different classes. In 2012, a young man who undergoes routine HIV testing and is detected early, and who has access to health care, lives a healthy lifestyle, and adheres to his regimen of HIV medications, can expect to live a full life. My colleague Sean Cahill and I recently wrote about this in *The Huffington Post* (Halkitis & Cahill, 2011), suggesting: "In 1981, a 20-year-old diagnosed with AIDS could expect to die from AIDS-related complications by age 22; today a newly diagnosed 20-year-old who adheres to treatment can expect to live well into his 50's and likely longer."

In the midst of these circumstances, there is also a group of men, men of my generation, who, despite the odds, despite the fact that they were infected prior to these medical advances, have managed to survive this plague, the true long-term survivors who managed to stay alive until 1996, the turning point in the AIDS epidemic, when combination antiviral treatment, first named HAART (highly active antiretroviral therapy, and now simply ART), radically shifted the course of the epidemic (Palella et al., 1998, 2006). The story of AIDS is thus also the story of these men. These long-term survivors diagnosed in a time of little hope have managed not only to survive but also to have reached middle age.

And now as these true long-term survivors enter middle age and older adulthood, the senior years in which they too can have an AARP card, there is no doubt a period of reflection on what has been and what lies ahead. Many of these men prepared for the deaths of those around them and their own deaths when they were in their 20s, 30s, and 40s. But they did not die. The *Miami Herald* recently reported about the graying of this AIDS Generation, indicating, "Once resigned to die, the afflicted get older" (Walker, 2011, p. 5A), and in a powerful op-ed in *The New York Times* (2011), Mark Trautwein described his living with AIDS as "the death sentence that defined my life." What must it be like to make it to this point and to this age, only to realize that now, truly, and based on normal estimates of life expectancy, the end is most certainly within sight? How do these men negotiate this reality of aging with a lifetime of expected death? Their stories of survival and resilience must be told as a testament to the gay men of my generation—those of us who now enter our golden years and those who never will. These stories are the stories of all of us, living or not.

Redirecting My Perspective on the AIDS Epidemic

In Jonathan Larson's Pulitzer Prize–winning musical *Rent*, which centers on a group of East Village, New York City, residents living and dying in the age of AIDS, one character describes his attempt to control the epidemic with his mind. For me, in many ways, my career in the world of HIV behavioral research has been directed by an attempt to intellectualize something that cannot be controlled physically. Through my science and my research, I have been able to create some reason around the chaos of the epidemic: "In the midst of the tragedy of AIDS and the deaths of many close to me, I was able to cope with the reality of the epidemic by intellectually managing it through research. It is the idea of mind over matter. And I hope that in that process of intellectualizing, we have enacted work that has a beneficial effect" (Halkitis & Marino, 2011, p. 17).

What I have come to know as I too now approach my middle age is that to move forward, I must move beyond the past. I am at this point of inflection. The stories of my loved ones have driven me for two decades. It is time to release them. It is time to take stock of those who still live—those who, like me, contribute to the fabric of the AIDS Generation.

Documenting the Life Experience of Long-Term Survivors

In this work, I document the life experiences of gay men who are long-term survivors of AIDS. I tell their battle stories from the last 30 years, share their views with the world as they emerge into their later stages of life, and, most importantly, document the strategies they applied to survive. In the end, I hope that through the words and stories of these men, I will demonstrate the resilience of my generation of gay men—the AIDS Generation.

I bring to this manuscript close to 20 years of behavioral research on gay men and HIV. I have interviewed and surveyed countless gay men, and what I have learned from them shapes my thinking in this volume. One program of research, however, is the one that most informs this work. It is a qualitative, ethnographic study that provides the rich data for this volume.

Between 2010 and 2012, my research team and I at the Center for Health, Identity, Behavior and Prevention Studies (CHIBPS) at NYU enacted a program of study involving aging HIV-positive men. The work emerged, as do many of our studies, from our ongoing dialogue about the impact of the AIDS epidemic in the United States, from our observation of the men in our world, and from the stories we had heard from the men we studied and within our own social circles. What became clear is that the life stories of gay men ages 50 and over who are long-term survivors of AIDS had to be told.

The program of inquiry, which we named Project Gold, implemented a methodological design that utilized in-depth exploratory interview techniques but, in addition, gathered data on behaviors and psychological states. While we sought to document the life experiences of these men who had survived AIDS, we also were as interested in understanding the struggles that older gay men face with their disease, the complications of aging in their lives, and how the health care system was meeting or failing to meet their needs.

Project Gold was enacted in two phases. In Phase I, we recruited a sample of 100 men, half current substance (i.e., drug) users and half nonusers, although the latter could have previously used substances. The overriding goal of the work was to test a theory of syndemics (Halkitis, Wolitski, & Millett, 2013) in this population—to determine the extent to which substance use, sex risk, and mental health burden are mutually reinforcing epidemics predisposed by psychosocial burdens including victimization and stigma (Halkitis, Kupprat, et al., 2013). The theory, which has garnered much attention in the field of HIV behavioral research (e.g., Halkitis, 2010a; Stall, Friedman, & Catania, 2008), had not been applied to a population of aging HIV-positive gay men. The sample was recruited through a variety of in-person and online outreach methods. Using targeted sampling, we oversampled men of color, given the prevalence of HIV in this segment of the population. In Phase II, we recruited an additional 100 men, regardless of substance use.

In both Phase I and II, the study participants were assessed via a quantitative survey, which was identical for both phases other than the addition of measures of spirituality and religiosity in Phase II. In Phase II the men also underwent testing for sexually transmitted infections (STIs)—genital, oral, and rectal gonorrhea as well as genital and rectal *Chlamydia*—to serve as proxy indicators of sexual risk taking and to determine if the men's health providers were adhering to recommended CDC guidelines for STI testing.

We conducted in-depth exploratory interviews of the 100 men for Phase I of Project Gold. The exploratory interviews sought to explicate the theory of syndemics but also to examine the life experiences of these aging

HIV-positive men, in relation to living with HIV and with regard to the process of aging. In Phase II the qualitative interview was replaced by a slightly modified exploratory interview that sought to document the experiences of trauma over the men's lifetimes. These data were gathered by members of my research team at CHIBPS.

Of the 200 men who participated in Project Gold, the majority were long-term survivors, most of whom were diagnosed with HIV/AIDS in the 1980s (between 1981 and 1989) and who were young men ages 18 to 32 at the time of their diagnoses. At the time of their interviews, they ranged in age from 50 to 61 and were diverse in terms of race/ethnicity—21% White, 38% Black, 5% Asian, 5% mixed race, and 31% Hispanic.

Thematic coding was used to analyze the initial set of interviews collected as part of Project Gold. This analytic process informed the structure for this volume. In this process, the main ideas regarding the volume emerged and directed the topics that are addressed in the ensuing chapters. The eight main themes that emerged from the analyses (i.e., the topics addressed in Chapter 3 through Chapter 6) were further specified by subthemes. Although I will draw from this initial set of interviews throughout the discourse as a means of forwarding the ideas and will utilize elements of this data set, the main ideas and voices presented in the book are drawn from a new set of in-depth interviews that I personally conducted with a set of 15 men who are gay long-term survivors of AIDS—the AIDS Generation interviews. Like Robert, Jim, Tony, Rick, and Cameron, these 15 long-term survivors came to know their lives as HIV-positive men in their young adulthood, at what should have been the peak of their lives. But unlike my five men who succumbed to the ravages of AIDS, these long-term survivors were still alive to tell their stories as middle-aged men.

The structure of the AIDS Generation interviews was shaped and informed by the preliminary work we conducted for Project Gold. These original interviews from Project Gold provided the foundation for the work, which was then more fully and completely explored in the interviews of the 15 men who are my representatives of the AIDS Generation. In the 15 interviews, questions were directly posed about the topics of each chapter and the data were then fully analyzed. *The AIDS Generation* is thus informed by the life experiences of a large number of men, with 15 voices, experiences, and stories reflected fully in the volume.

The interviews with the men of the AIDS Generation examined how HIV and AIDS shaped the physical, emotional, and social lives of these men; how these long-term survivors coped with the illness in the absence of any effective treatments; and how these men understand and cope with the aging process as they emerge into the later stages of life. The purpose of the interviews was to document behaviors of these men throughout the course of the last 30 years to examine and delineate strategies for survival, which may be indicative of resilience. This work is also of critical importance given that the life experiences of these men are unique to a generation, given the rapid evolution of treatments for HIV and the transformation of HIV to a chronic disease. Current generations of gay men, while still experiencing this health disparity, are not subject to the decimation and death that was experienced by the AIDS Generation.

My approach to the qualitative data analysis of these 15 men's life stories was directed by multiple approaches to qualitative data analysis but relies heavily on one particular orientation. For the purposes of examining the data, I have applied the tenets of both grounded theory and thematic coding. However, in listening to and reading the stories, I sought to dig deeper, to look beyond the words, and to place myself in the life experiences of these men. I examined more than just what was said, seeking an inner voice, inspired by my colleague and friend Carol Gilligan. My primary approach to the data utilizes the innovative and state-of-the-art methodology known as the *Listening Guide Method of Psychological Inquiry* (Gilligan, Spencer, Weinberg, & Bertsch, 2003), a discovery-based qualitative component that was employed to delineate strategies for survival evidenced in the lives of the long-term survivors. Like Gilligan, whose transformative work *In a Different Voice* (1993) sought to understand and delineate the development of women using their own voices and, in turn, to de-pathologize the development of women, which had been directed for years by a male-dominated profession and male-constructed paradigms, my goal is to de-pathologize the lives and developmental processes of gay men, and in particular the lives of aging HIV-positive men who have survived an epidemic and have demonstrated power and resilience. Using this lens for analysis, I seek to correct "problems" or "deficits" that the behavioral literature has often associated with gay men in general and HIV-positive gay men in particular. Moreover, I seek to correct misconceptions of gay men that still permeate vast segments of the American consciousness and finally to show that the AIDS epidemic was not a sign of our "weakness" but a test of our strength.

My Stance—The Power of Seropositive Gay Men

Throughout the course of history, gay men have been labeled as effeminate and weak. Sissy men could not be "real" men, after all. Driven by research dominated by primarily heterosexual society, gay men's behavior was seen as deviant and as a sign of both emotional and physical weakness. This conception perpetuated our American consciousness for decades and was portrayed in the media by characters who were not openly gay but obviously gay—Paul Lynde's Uncle Arthur in *Bewitched*, for example, or Tony Randall's Felix in *The Odd Couple*. After all, a gay man could not be emotionally grounded or masculine—these were attributes confined to the heterosexual men. It must have been challenging for heterosexual America when their manliest of men, Rock Hudson, turned out to be both gay and suffering from AIDS, and who ultimately died on October 3, 1985 (Berger, 1985).

Unfortunately, with the onset of AIDS, the conception of gay men as fragile and weak was manifested in our physical beings. I have written about this matter previously and have shown that the AIDS epidemic helped to perpetuate the stereotype that the heterosexual world had imposed upon us (Halkitis, 1999, 2001). For all the advances that the AIDS epidemic brought forward in medicine, in our thinking about public health and infectious disease, in the development of approval of pharmaceuticals, and in community organizing, it simultaneously created a condition for gay men where the 10 steps we had taken forward in the 1970s in asserting our civil rights were followed by 30 steps back. I believe we are only now beginning to recover from that setback.

Sadly, like all AIDS-related deaths, Rock Hudson's death was tragic, but it also functioned as a catalyst in realigning the cognitive schema some were using to understand gay men. It is this schema that I seek to further modify with this manuscript, as we begin to envision gay men using a model of resilience rather than a model of deficit through the actions of the AIDS Generation.

Thus, there is one very clear objective I hope to achieve in this work. The goal of this book is to share the lived experiences of gay men who are long-term survivors of AIDS as powerful and strong—to show that the lived experiences of these men are stories of determination, power, and, above all, resilience—the characteristics often attributed to and reserved for heterosexuals but that are much more evident in the manner in which seropositive gay men have managed their lives. I will examine the words these men use as an indicator of how they see the world and see themselves in the world, and, most importantly, how they navigated and made sense of a world in which AIDS was destroying everything they knew and loved and were promised after the Stonewall Riots of 1969. In other words, I will give voice to experiences that, to date, have not fully been heard.

This work seeks to be more than simply descriptive and anecdotal. It is an ethnographic analysis of coping strategies and systems for surviving. Underlying the delineation of these life experiences of HIV-positive gay long-term survivors is the notion that we, in particular those who provide health services and care, can learn from the experiences of these men. From their experiences, and the manner in which gay long-term survivors of HIV have managed their lives, one can glean a better understanding of resilience. Such knowledge would help not only to inform working with a new generation that is affected by and infected with HIV but also to assist those living with other demanding and chronic diseases. As recently noted in *The New York Times* (Considine, 2011), referring to HIV-positive men as they enter middle age, "There are many people who are survivors, and who have tremendous resilience, of course."

Throughout this volume, I will purposely intertwine and complement these lived experiences within the historical contexts. I will draw upon the extant academic literature from the last 30 years and from the writings in the popular press and will infuse references to the small yet powerful collective of artistic works addressing AIDS to capture the reality in the early days of the epidemic. Thus, throughout the manuscript, which will rely most on the interviews I conducted, I will also interweave these elements to support or further illuminate and realize the life experiences of the men with whom we spoke.

Finally, beyond any academic role this book may play in helping to advance science, I simply want to celebrate the lives of gay men who, despite all logic and reason and without any hope at the time of their diagnosis, are long-term survivors of AIDS—my generation, the AIDS Generation, the bravest generation—in determination that our stories will not be forgotten.

CHAPTER 2 | ## The Men of the AIDS Generation
A Study of Gay Men Surviving AIDS

RALPH, ONE OF THE men of the AIDS Generation who you will come to know in this chapter, described his life living with HIV, including through the darkest moments and times of little hope, as follows:

> Our experiences write our history and so I, um, think without these experiences I wouldn't have been or become who I am now, and so although I didn't really enjoy it, I appreciate it.

Between April and June of 2012, interviews were conducted with 15 men, all HIV-positive, all gay, ranging in age from 40 to 58, and all long-term survivors of AIDS. The interviews were conducted in my office at NYU with windows on two sides overlooking Washington Square Park to the west and the Brown Building, the site of the infamous Triangle Shirt Factory fire, to the north. Each year on the anniversary of that tragic fire—a public health nightmare—a ceremony is conducted, and at the conclusion of this public acknowledgment, a standing arrangement of flowers is placed alongside the plaque on the Brown Building. This annual recognition is a testament to the lives of those, mostly young immigrant women, who perished on that day in 1912. A mile away, the beauty of the 9/11 Memorial provides a place of comfort and refection regarding those who lost their lives on that infamous day. It struck me more than once during the course of these interviews, with the former World Trade Center site just south of my office and the Brown Building right across the street, that no true place of mourning exists for those who have lost their lives to the AIDS disaster, although recent efforts have been undertaken to create the AIDS Memorial Park on the grounds of the former St. Vincent's Hospital in Greenwich Village.

A maroon leather-like sofa was situated on the south side of the office so that each man could look out onto the surrounding environment during the course of the interview. I sat on a chair adjacent to the couch with my back to the western windows, and a small table was placed in front of the sofa where we could rest our bottled waters, coffees, and other beverages during the course of the conversation. At first, I had placed a box of tissues on the table, but recognizing the potentially leading nature of this gesture, I placed the tissues on my desk behind my chair and only moved the box to the table during the interviews when there was a need. More often than not, I reached for the tissues.

Originally, I had planned to interview only 10 men, but as these interviews were being conducted, I realized the complexity of the task that was in front of me. Because the men with whom I spoke came from all walks of life, from various cultural backgrounds, from diverse means and circumstances, of different sizes and shapes, the stories of their lives as HIV-positive gay men were also widely differing. My instinct was thus to speak with more rather than fewer men, believing that my understanding of these life experiences would be more fully realized from a larger sample. In retrospect I also believe that my desire to spend time with more of these men was driven by a sense of kinship and connection—my peers whose life experiences evolved in tandem with my own evolution into middle age.

Throughout the interviews there was an immediate connection and camaraderie with my peers, men of my generation who had lived through the very dark years of the AIDS epidemic. Like me, all were approaching or had emerged into middle age, with a lifetime of loss and sorrow. The connection with each of the men was immediate. There was no awkwardness or any sense on the men's part that I was a dispassionate academic studying a population I knew very little about; rather, there was the sense that I was one of them—a peer, a brother, a fellow warrior. Ralph expressed this idea clearly to me: "It's interesting that, you know, it's not like, um, you can't relate to any of this, that you're just hearing it. It's great that you're asking me the same stuff that you could probably answer." And he was correct. Often when the men cried during the interviews, so did I. Our experiences and our lives were bonded by the AIDS crisis.

Finding the Men

For anyone who has conducted behavioral research, the task of recruiting study participants can be a harrowing one, especially if the subject matter of the research addresses issues of risk such as substance use and sexual risk taking. Well-intentioned researchers conducting work with gay men have struggled with this element of their studies, failing often to recognize that humans are savvy, that gay men are sophisticated, and that for many a monetary incentive is irrelevant. What many of these men want is to be heard, to be respected, and to contribute to a program of study that might ameliorate the blow of the AIDS epidemic in their community. They can see through researchers who are not well intentioned, and they know more than most groups how to work around the system.

Recruiting men for Project Gold, the research work that laid the foundation for this book, and for the book project proved to be a relatively easy task. Both phases of Project Gold, which included a sample of 200 men, took only 5 months to complete (Halkitis, Kupprat, et al., 2013), and many of the men who participated in the research project expressed awe and surprise at the fact that we wanted to "study" them. After years of being prodded and poked, filling endless vials with their own blood, being swabbed, and being scanned, the men who participated both in our preliminary work and in the AIDS Generation interviews just wanted to be heard. For many of the men, the experience of being interviewed and asked questions about their lives was an honor and point of reflection. When asked to describe himself, Eddie, one of the 15, said,

> Wow. Um, actually, I love that question. I was asked—asked that question, um, several years ago and I was homeless and, um, trying to get into a shelter. And, um, I wasn't sure exactly what to tell them, but now I do.

For all 15 men, there has been a lifetime of reflection, of wondering, of considering, and this was an opportunity to tell their stories.

Recruitment of the men whose stories you will come to know in this volume was undertaken by my team. Unlike large-scale quantitative studies that require systematized and overconstructed sampling paradigms to ensure generalizability of results and the power of our analytic procedures, we were motivated by identifying men who could effectively share their life experiences and also whose lived experiences represented different aspects and realties of the HIV/AIDS epidemic for the last 30 years. In such historical accounts as in recent documentary films such as David

France's powerful *How to Survive a Plague*, one often learns about the experiences of upper middle- and middle-class White men, engaged in activism, and with social capital that empowered them to survive. Certainly this is one take of AIDS, but we sought more than these experiences. In that regard, we cast the net widely, both drawing on the men who participated in Project Gold and reaching out through near-peer and electronic and social networks (e.g., Strength in Number [SIN] New York City) to recruit our sample.

The study team screened all of the men who were interviewed. Our criteria for inclusion were prescribed but somewhat wide in scope. These criteria included being a gay man diagnosed with HIV or AIDS prior to the implementation of highly active antiretroviral therapy (HAART) in 1996, approaching or in the middle-age period of life (40 to 60 years old), and being a young adult at the time of diagnosis. Using these parameters, we were able to identify gay men who were first aware of their status in the 1980s and early 1990s before any truly effective treatment was available. Because our focus was on gay men, we did not apply the Centers for Disease Control and Prevention (CDC) epidemiological and behavioral criterion of "men who have sex with men" (MSM), which ultimately undermines the well-being of my population (Halkitis, 2010a), but rather men who were firmly situated in their sexual identities as gay. The story of *The AIDS Generation* is the story of gay men.

Sandy, Francesca, Jessica, and Molly, my research assistants, provided potential participants with information about the book project, which was approved by the NYU Committee on Activities Involving Human Subjects (i.e., institutional review board). Men were also screened for eligibility criteria and were asked to provide a brief description of their lives as HIV-positive gay men. Based on these initial conversations, the interviews were scheduled for 2-hour blocks of time at my office on Washington Square.

On the day of his scheduled interview, each man was greeted in the lobby of my office building by one of the research assistants. Each was escorted to my office where I welcomed him, and then undertook the consent process with the assigned research assistant. Of note is the fact that all of the men arrived on time or early and on the occasion; when one was delayed due to subway congestion, he called to inform us of the situation.

At first, most of the participants appeared hesitant in their approach with me. This was perhaps due to a perceived power differential or because they were entering the hallowed walls of NYU to take part in a study. Perhaps it was due to their uncertainty and potential anxiety in recalling their life stories, or because they were uncertain on how I would approach this work. However, any anxiety quickly dissipated as I explained to each my own stories of loss in the age of AIDS, grappling with my oncoming middle age, and my desire to write the book to honor the men of our generation. To Hal I explained the purpose of my work, as I did to the other study participants, as follows:

> I've been in HIV behavioral research for the last 15 years, the last couple of years really focusing a lot of attention on older positive gay men, and decided that one of the things I really wanted to do in addition to the research is give voice to our generation of men and what we've been through... and how resilient we are and to celebrate us. And so I put together a book proposal.... So I am in the process, and you are, as you heard from Francesca, number six I'm talking to. I'm going to speak with 15, maybe 20 men... and then sort of put it together for a book that's going be called *The AIDS Generation*. So during the course of our conversation today we'll just talk about a variety of things, whatever you feel comfortable talking about or that you want to share with me.

The Interview

The qualitative data of Project Gold informed the development of the interview protocol. The protocol, as originally conceived, was semi-structured in nature, allowing for maximum flexibility in the data collection such that the men with whom I spoke could share their stories and experiences. Eight main themes or life experiences were explored: (1) the initial diagnosis with HIV or HIV/AIDS, (2) loss due to the epidemic, (3) strategies for survival in the absence of effective treatments, (4) both active and avoidant coping strategies to deal with the epidemic including the use of substances and sex as means of coping, (5) activism and community building in the AIDS era, (6) the breakthrough of effective therapies in 1996 and the aftermath of these advances, (7) aging as a gay HIV-positive man, and (8) understandings of survival. For each of these themes, I developed a set of probe questions to explore the concepts more fully.

Throughout the discourse with each participant, these main themes were explored, although not in a linear or an overly prescribed fashion. I centered each interview on each man, allowing him to relay his stories, experiences, and understandings in the manner with which he was most comfortable, and to use his own logic to relay the ideas and make sense of the events in his life. Although my goal was to explore each of the domains, these explorations varied from participant to participant. As a result, each session was a conversation, a natural discourse between two men, rather than a data collection session driven by the agenda of the researcher. The questions and probes sat face down on the table. Not once did I turn to these probing questions, and by the fifth interview I realized that these questions that were placed on the table, at first as reassurance and backup for me, were not required.

My questions, when posed, sought to clarify and define and to seek a deeper meaning in the words the men were using to fully understand the thoughts and logic associated with their words, how they understood these words, and the meanings associated with the words on cognitive and socio-emotional levels. A typical interaction is shown below:

EDDIE: And what I do on a daily basis is make sure that I represent who I know I am.
PERRY: Which is will?
EDDIE: Which is will. Wisdom, integrity, and love.
PERRY: What do you mean by wisdom, integrity, and love?

This approach to the interview process necessitated that I release my agenda, focus on every word each man shared and every sentence that was uttered, and reflect on what was being said and how messages were conveyed. This process, as I explained to the participants, would create a situation that had the feeling of a conversation, a discussion between two peers who are sharing life events. In that regard, I too shared from my life during the course of the conversation, demonstrating my own vulnerabilities and struggles as a gay man who came of age as part of the AIDS Generation. After Richard, another of the 15, described his first sexual experience with a man in which he expressed terror, his uneasiness in retelling that event was apparent. To diffuse this unsettled feeling and to support the sense that he was not alone in such experiences and feelings, I interjected as follows:

So at 18, something similar happens to me. I drop off my girlfriend at the time from a date, and I'm walking on the way back home to my parents' house in Queens. I don't know how I know this, but some guy tries to pick me up. We end up going to his apartment. There's lots of kissing and making out and sucking. And I'm terrified, right, for the next 3 weeks. And this is a month—the month before I have to go to college in Columbia in the big bad city across the river.

This approach to the collection of data resulted in narratives that were each unique—15 idiosyncratic stories and experiences that gave voice to each of the men with whom I spoke, that celebrated the life of each man, empowering each to share his tales with me with no fear of being reduced to a point of datum, a unit of analysis. From the perspective of a traditional social science research and analytic paradigm, the end product—the data—was much more challenging to analyze, making it more difficult to determine commonalities and themes that cut across the experiences. However, the data were also more honest and true to the experiences of the men, thus outweighing the often rigid and prescribed approach to the collection of narrative data that results in disconnected, fragmented stories that lack meaning. Meaning making ultimately was the goal of this work, and the approach that I applied allowed me to achieve this goal and directed me to attend to the narratives rather than my own agenda.

Carol Gilligan describes her approach to her work on the moral development of women as "grounded in listening" (1993, p. xiii). Like Gilligan, I sought to listen to how each of the men explained and described his life living with HIV. I listened for how each spoke of himself as a gay man, as an aging man, as an HIV-positive man, and how each understood the intersection of these identities—an aging, gay, HIV-positive man. I also listened for how each man negotiated the traumas of living with HIV at a time when the disease was considered, and in fact was, a death sentence; living as a gay man coming of age when the gay rights movement was only in its infancy; and living as an older man in a culture obsessed with youth and virility. How did these men negotiate their lives in their young adulthood when they first were diagnosed with HIV? How did they experience their lives as young men who had to attend to the realities of a chronic viral infection that weakened their bodies and aged them rapidly? How did their HIV status direct their lives? How do they understand the perpetuation of the HIV epidemic in now three generations of gay men? Mostly, I listened for how each man understood his survival after living with HIV for 20 to 30 years.

The approach to data collection also allowed me to develop a camaraderie and kinship with these men—my peers—who have lived through the realities of the AIDS epidemic from the very onset in the 1980s. These life experiences bonded us, our developmental stage and ages created a connection, and the experiences of pain we shared created a sense of relief from retelling these stories with someone who truly and deeply understood the often-painful and debilitating events in our lives. Ultimately, what bonded us most was the mystery of why we were in that office at New

York University (NYU) together when so many of those we knew had lost their voices and their lives during the last three decades. The experience for me was encapsulated perfectly by Michael Callen (1990, p. 21), who describes the interviews he undertook with long-term survivors in the first decade of AIDS with the following powerful statement: "As long-term survivors began to crawl out of the woodworks, I realized that before I interviewed them, I'd have to come up with a list of questions. In order to do that, I would have to do some soul-searching: Why did I think I was still alive?" During every interview this statement and sentiment came to my mind and served as a reminder that the journey I was embarking upon was profound and significant, and that unlike Michael Callen, I had been afforded the opportunity to be interviewing these powerful men in 2012, when AIDS as an immediate death sentence had become a thing of the past. It also reminded me of the interviews we conducted at the onset of my career as an HIV behavioral researcher and the number of those men we had interviewed who had since perished (Halkitis, Gomez, & Wolitksi, 2005). Mostly this work helped me to focus on my own values. My life was changed during the time when I interacted with these men and wrote about their spectacular lives.

It was also apparent that the approach I used was unfamiliar to some of the men who previously had participated in research studies or who were research savvy. This created uneasiness for some in their roles as research participants, as noted most clearly at the conclusion of the interview with Ralph:

> Well, I would hope to think that the information I have given you is something that I would like to be representative of who I am, but you know, what I told you I'm sure there's a hundred million things in my head that I wish I would have said. I mean, I'm happy with what I told you, but, um, I hope I didn't delete or not say anything about things that I feel are important and need to be said.

Ralph's statement also underscores the degree to which the men of the AIDS Generation understood and experienced this project as an opportunity to share their stories. They need to be heard—fully heard.

The Analysis

Each of the 15 interviews was transcribed by an agency we had subcontracted. When the interviews were returned to us, the transcripts were reconciled with the digital recordings by the research team to check for accuracy. Corrections were manually made in the transcripts of words and terms, which might have been lost in transcription because the word processors (both person and software) were unfamiliar with the jargon being used by the study participant.

My approach to the interviews was highly personal. Not only did I conduct the interviews and observe the men as they sat across from me retelling their stories, but I also reimmersed myself in the conversation on several occasions over the course of several months, both by rereading the transcripts and examining the words with my eyes and by relistening to the interviews and examining the words with my ears. I purposely reexamined the interviews in varying orders, at different times of day, and in different environments, opening myself up to the possibility that something new would emerge in my reviewing of the "data." As I listened to the interviews, I closed my eyes on many occasions, visualizing the actual interview, what each man was wearing, where he was sitting, how he looked or didn't look at me as we spoke, how he reacted to my questions, when he fidgeted, when he cried, and when there was a break or a change in his voice. Most of the men also provided me with electronic photos of themselves, which I kept open on the desktop during the writing process.

As I indicated in Chapter 1, I did not utilize any one particular approach to the analysis of the interview, although the ethos of this work was highly influenced by the work of Carol Gilligan. In 1993, Gilligan wrote a Letter to Readers, as a prelude to her volume *In a Different Voice*, in which she states (p. xii), "In the years since *In a Different Voice* was published, many people have spoken to me about their lives, their marriages, their divorces, their work, their relationships, and their children. . . . Their experiences, their examples of different voices, and their ideas expand and complicate what I have written, often in highly creative ways." This sentence is powerful and meaningful to me. The interviews that I have conducted have pushed me to think in a more expansive manner about the task in front of me.

As I embarked on the writing of this work, I had somewhat clear notions about what I wanted to write. I had a prescribed table of contents, which I had proposed based on the thematic coding of data from Project Gold. Topics and themes had emerged from these original data that provided me with a very clear outline for the format of what I wanted to write. In fact, in the ensuing chapters, these themes from Project Gold are explored as a means of framing each of the topics. And although I remain true to this original structure, what has evolved over the course of the interviews and the readings is my approach to conveying the findings from the interviews of the 15 men. Rather than simply retelling events and stories and quantifying emerging themes, I attempt instead to share each man's voice in relation to the topics addressed in this book. For example, while conveying how each man first found out about his HIV status, I of course attend to the circumstances and contexts of this monumental event, but attend equally to how each man tells this story, how he conveys the information, and his emotional state in sharing this event in his life—to his voice.

My approach to the analysis of the 15 interviews is radically different from the one my colleagues and I used in our edited volume, *HIV + Sex: The Psychological and Interpersonal Dynamic of HIV-Seropositive Gay and Bisexual Men's Relationships* (Halkitis, Gomez, et al., 2005, p. 10), where we utilized a quantitative analysis software and described our analyses to the qualitative data that constitute the book, as follows: "Authors of individual chapters began their analyses with the pre-coded data set. In most instances, the authors organized their analyses around a limited number of standardized interview questions or used the presence of global codes to identify relevant responses regardless of where they appeared in the interview." I cite this example of my previous work not as a means of commenting on any shortcomings. That was a very different type of work, directed primarily by positivist paradigm. The product was powerful but very different from the approach and my goal in this book. At the conclusion of each interview for this current book, I provided each man with a copy of the edited volume, which many of them asked me to sign. My purpose was to share with each man a personal token but also to provide a framework for the current project in which his story would be depicted. I explained this to Eddie as follows:

So I'm going to give you my card and I'm also going to give you a copy of a book that I wrote in the late '90s, which is just kind of like stories of positive men, but it's kind of—it's not like the book I'm going write, but it is to give you a flavor of the book that I'm going to write.

Approximately 3 months after the interviews were completed, we gathered the men as a group for a follow-up discussion. Twelve of the 15 attended, and the meeting, which took the format of a focus group, sought to clarify some of the issues that emerged from the individual interviews and provide an opportunity for the participants to share their stories and their experiences with each other. Specifically, we examined two main issues— strategies for survival and the process of aging. I was also directed by a desire to examine each man's voice within the context of a group of peers, building on the voice I had heard in the one-on-one interviews. Finally, I wanted to provide a venue for the men to meet each other and to celebrate each other. This gathering was also inspired by the thoughts of one of the men, Kerry, who clearly articulated the need for a space for older HIV-positive gay men to meet each other outside the context of a support group or a social gathering in bar: "Maybe it should be more like, not like necessarily the T Dance, but maybe there should be a function or something that people can socialize at regularly. Even if it were once a month or something." For 2 beautiful hours, we sat together, talked, cried, and shared ideas and experiences.

These 2 hours we spent together created a new "band of brothers." Each man demonstrated great respect for his peers, and many wiped tears from their eyes as they shared their life stories. Each attended to the comments of the others, rarely interrupting, and always listening and reflecting on the words of the others. In my years conducting focus groups such as this one, I was required to manage and coordinate the efforts of the group. In this case, my oversight was limited only to keeping us on schedule because it was clear at the end of the 2 hours that this session could have been extended to 4 or 6 hours given the level of engagement.

At the conclusion, all of the men exchanged names, e-mail addresses, and other contact information to stay in touch with each other. Their camaraderie was natural and easy and simply beautiful to witness, and many exchanges have taken place within this group. This session was also digitally recorded and transcribed, and elements of that conversation are utilized throughout the course of the volume. When I do draw from this conversation, I purposely retain the interjections of others while one of the men was speaking to demonstrate the dynamics in the room.

Post–focus group and throughout the writing of this volume, I also have been in electronic communication with the men. My communications were undertaken via e-mail when I confronted a passage of text in the interview or focus group that required further clarification. In every instance the man to whom the question was posed responded almost immediately. On three other occasions I posed a question to the entire group and asked the men to react and reflect on an idea I was considering. Again, elements of these correspondences are included in this volume.

The Men of the AIDS Generation

In the chapters that follow you will come to know the 15 men, the long-term survivors and their stories. Their words are unadulterated as the thoughts and the voices of each man are shared. The narratives are never blended to create composite characters so as to enhance the effect of the work. In other words, the story of each man stands on its own, blemishes and all, with utterances, and stammering, and pauses in thought so each reader can fully experience the realities of each man. The only modification made has been to the name of each of the participants and their close relations, and a limited amount of other identifying information that could reveal who they are in order to respect their privacies.

At the end of each interview and after each man had departed, I reflected on the interview and commented directly into the digital recorder. These reflections were my immediate reactions to the interview that had just concluded. I allowed myself to express freely about the interview, the stories that were shared, and my own personal reaction to each man. Thereafter and based on my repeated readings and listenings, I came to my own knowing of each man.

Early in my graduate education, I was introduced to the *Up Series* British documentaries, the first of which was made in 1964 by Granada Television and was named *7 Up*. The series has lasted for 49 years, following a group of 14 British children from age 7 and every 7 years thereafter (*56 Up* was released in January 2013). The major thesis of this work is informed by the Jesuit saying "Give me a child until he is seven and I will give you the man." This understanding of human development is one that also has highly influenced my own work and thinking throughout the last two decades. Thus, in describing the 15 men who are members of the AIDS Generation, I provide some key demographic information for each and then delve into their childhood stories—who they were as children, or, more accurately, how they retell the stories of their lives as children. I come to understand the lives of these HIV-positive gay men and their lifelong experiences, their survival, and their resilience through the lens of their formative years in childhood and adolescence. The lives of these men as children often shape their adult lives with HIV.

Ralph

For Ralph, a 53-year-old Latino man, who has a striking resemblance to Queen front man Freddy Mercury, the experience of AIDS for his generation of gay men is akin to the Holocaust: "Like the Holocaust, it was our own personal little holocaust, and we had to go from where we lived into the ghetto, being San Francisco." In fact, as an adult gay man living with

AIDS, Ralph found himself drawn to the concentration camps of World War II: "I've been to the ghettos too. But I've been to Auschwitz." For Ralph, the experience of HIV is complicated by coinfection with hepatitis C, compromising his health to an even greater extent.

A mother born in Texas to Mexican immigrants and a father of German French extraction raised Ralph in Salt Lake City, in a family of seven children. Despite being raised Catholic, Ralph describes his upbringing as informed by Mormonism, which he views as having had a favorable impact on his life: "Mormon was definitely an influence because everybody was Mormon....I have to give credit to those horrible people because their influence is probably what kept me away from drugs and alcohol when I was a kid." In the focus group, Ralph described himself to the others as follows:

> I'm Ralph. I was diagnosed—I'm not sure of the date. I actually don't remember the date. I just remember the experience though. But I'm guessing early '80s. I'm gonna be 54 in October. I like to round up these days. just seems a lot easier than rounding down like it used to be. [Ralph laughs] I've been living in New York for maybe 15 years, San Francisco for 15 years before that. And I became HIV-positive in Utah, so that was a kinda scary place to have that happen. Quickly moved to California.

In fact, Ralph worked as a bartender on Castro Street in San Francisco at the height of the epidemic.

Throughout the course of the interview, Ralph was very concerned about doing and saying "the right thing," seeking to please me with his narratives. He relied heavily on his self-understanding as someone who is not very intelligent but who had to rely on his looks, despite the fact that he was poised and articulate and insightful throughout the course of the interview. When I pushed back and commented on his perception of his own intelligence, he shied away and lost eye contact with me. Ralph attributes his lack of intellectual achievement to his parents, indicating, "I had lousy parents who never really motivated me...."

Repeatedly, Ralph described how he depended heavily on his looks throughout the course of his life and believed that any successes were tied to his appearance. In his older age, he has become less self-assured in this regard, sadly suggesting that sexual partners are disappointed when they meet him. Interestingly, despite a lifelong reliance on looks, Ralph now scorns the fact that many in the gay community judge by appearance, and thus immerses himself in contexts where he judges his looks at the higher end of the spectrum. Speaking of a specific social gathering of gay men, Ralph said: "I think that group of people is less attractive and for some reason that's more comfortable for me."

Antoine

When asked to describe himself, Antoine, who has been living with HIV since 1986, said, "Antoine is a 52-year-old African American man, who is actually gay, born this way, thank you." Like many of the other men, Antoine's recollection of his life as a gay man traces back to an early childhood age, although like the others, he could not articulate what he sensed or thought or believed at that time:

> I mean I—I can go back to honestly saying to you, I had my first gay thought at 4 years old, but I didn't know it was a gay thought. I knew I was gay in kindergarten when I raised my hand to ask my teacher to go to the bathroom because I wanted to look at the boy that was with my cousin, who was, I thought, who was just absolutely gorgeous.

This sensibility and sense of humor and love of life expressed in this comment were evident throughout our conversation, as Antoine spoke with great honor and respect for his life as a gay man growing up in Brooklyn, New York, and whose formative years and emerging adulthood were informed by the relationships he developed cruising for sex in Prospect Park, which he describes as "Mecca." This self-assuredness and confidence as a gay man is clearly fueled by the support and acceptance he experienced from his mother as young boy, who had passed away the year prior to the interview:

> ANTOINE: Because I believe my mom always knew. Because I used to state to her, no African American mom buys their son a Barbie doll record player at 7 years old for a Christmas present.
> PERRY: And she gave you that. Did you ask for that or—
> ANTOINE: No. She said because it was the last thing in the store, and she didn't want me to have—didn't, she didn't want me to not have anything for Christmas. And I'm like, "Okay, I can get past the, um, Barbie doll record player, but the first 45 you bought me was Aretha Franklin's I've Never Loved a Man the Way I Love You."
> PERRY: Mm-hm.
> ANTOINE: And I'm 8 years old.

PERRY: Mm-hm.

ANTOINE: [Laughs]. And at 15, when she asked—when I said to her that I was gay and that I would not make her any grandchildren, she said, "Oh, I already knew that. I was just waiting for you to catch up."

PERRY: Interesting. It's almost like she was giving you like permission with the record player.

ANTOINE: Yeah.

This self-confidence was evident as he spoke of his life living with HIV, including the support system he had with his circle of friends—his family he had developed as a young man in Prospect Park, who he refers to with terms associated with family relatives: "My gay mother was named Gene. My gay father was named Ronald, who was going to school to be an attorney. He was White. My gay aunt, Wilson, was a—how do you say it? He worked in a childcare agency." And at the same time he speaks with great sadness about his gay family, recalling the circle of 40 that constituted this family in 1985 and then reporting, "And right now, it's just me and Bianca," the rest having died of AIDS.

It also is evident in how he navigates social contexts, even when a colleague's homophobic husband questions Antoine's sexual orientation because of Antoine's depth of knowledge about sports. For Antoine, his survival and his ability to overcome the many challenges in his life are understood in terms of his sexual orientation. Antoine perceives that being gay was a source of power, which emboldened him to move beyond the established norms of the neighborhood and culture in which he was raised and which has led to a life of self-acceptance and contentment, first inspired by his mother and then by his gay family formed in Prospect Park. When asked how he feels about being an older HIV-positive gay man, Antoine smiled and said:

I'm loving it. I never thought it would be this wonderful. I'm comfortable with myself and I'm happy with my state of mind. And all the things that was once said to me that I couldn't do—and if it wasn't for the fact that I was gay and am gay, it would have never happened. I finished high school because I was gay. Because my straight friends didn't want to go to school, and when they said to me, "Why are you going to school?" I wrote down the word "bedroom," [and] two of them said, "bedrock." I said, "Yeah, that's why I go to school."

More than once during this initial interview with Antoine I was reminded of our brother, gay activist and educator Marlon Riggs, who died of AIDS complications in 1994, and his 1989 brilliant documentary about an African American gay man, *Tongues Untied.*

Gianni

Gianni was the first man interviewed in April 2012. He is 49 years old, the child of European immigrants, born and raised in the outskirts of Manhattan, New York. Gianni is highly educated, holding advanced graduate degrees. A self-made man, Gianni has Sylvester Stallone/John Travolta looks, works and speaks with confidence, and is highly knowledgeable about the medical aspects of HIV/AIDS. His approach to the disease is an intellectual one, and he relies on his cognition and logic to explain his AIDS journey, rarely allowing emotion and affect to enter his recollections, which he describes as compartmentalizing. Gianni was diagnosed with HIV/AIDS in 1988, although he traces his infection to 1981.

When Gianni speaks of his upbringing, the theme that emerges is one of control and management, skills he needed to develop as a young child because his parents assumed no responsibility other than housing and feeding him: "I mean, I've just been self-sufficient from a very young age," and despite these demands, he indicates, "And it's served me very well," suggesting that his life successes are directed in part by the expectations in his childhood.

Gianni describes his childhood as one where he was asked always to "be a man" as his parents navigated their new homeland with anxiety and apprehension. This condition persisted throughout his adolescence and as he prepared for college:

> I had to navigate figuring out how to pay for school 'cause my parents were useless. Had to get a student loan, had to get student, you know, uh, federal assistance, state—and which was different at that time. That's why I ended up paying nothing for college at the end of the day, but I had to do that on my own. Like I had to be the adult taking care of this stuff.

For Gianni, handling and managing these responsibilities in his childhood were not seen as an option but as an expectation: "I feel like everything in my life I've worked for myself." This approach of control and overmanagement in his life also informs how he subverted his sexuality throughout his adolescence:

> I didn't even know what to do about being gay, but I didn't—so here's the gay thing. So the gay thing was so I was pretty sure I was gay because I felt

attracted to men, but I did nothing about it all through high school because I didn't think I could because of where I was growing up and because I wanted to fit in. And because I wanted to go to prom and I wanted to have a girlfriend and I wanted to do what every other American boy was doing. Right. So and I had sex with women, and I don't know, that was fine, but I kind of knew something wasn't really all there for me with women. And it had gotten worse, like from 14 to 18 it got—it was sort of like this like drum—the way I can—I—I sense is that it was like this drum beat that got more and more and more intense the older I got.

Gianni's entire adult life is informed by AIDS, being infected during only his second sexual encounter with a man, and having lost three of his five boyfriends to the disease, one in his 20s, one in his 30s, and one in his 40s. Gianni, in fact, recalls the story of his infection in great detail and describes the death of Tom, the man he was involved with at the time, who had infected him, and whose death he witnessed as a 22-year-old in 1985:

Right, he had cancer, and that's what he died of. But I was pretty sure from what I had been reading at that point that it was AIDS. And, you know, I completely—I was petrified but completely suppressed it and didn't think about it because there was nothing I could really do at that point in time about it. But I knew in the back of my mind that I was probably positive.

In the last 5 years, Gianni has been married and indicates, "After all of this death and loss, I feel like I finally have the life I was hoping for at 20. AIDS really derailed all of that." During our interview, Gianni often used pop music to describe his feelings, as will be demonstrated in his statements throughout this volume.

Bobby and John

In the second week of April I interviewed Bobby and John, whose stories had become intertwined in the months that preceded the interviews. A romantic couple, Bobby and John spoke of their love for each other and their upcoming nuptials, despite the fact that they had only met each other within the last year.

Bobby, 47 years old, is a child of the Bayou who spent most of his formative years in Louisiana and describes his place of birth as "a poor Black town" (although he is White); he works as a special education teacher in the public school system of New York City. His work as a teacher may be connected to Bobby's love of school, which he recollects as he describes himself as child:

> I was an angel. I was never in trouble. I made more than straight A's. I said "yes, ma'am" and "no, sir" and I made my bed, well I wasn't so neat, but I ate and didn't talk back and I loved my homework and I loved my school. I was just a good, quiet kid. Never broke anything. I can tell you the five times I was in trouble in all of elementary school.

Bobby is tall, lean, and extremely handsome, and one is left to wonder how many heads he turned and hearts he broke in his lifetime. Bobby relied heavily on his sexuality to convey his stories, and his story of HIV/ AIDS was often nested within the context of sexuality and his own sobriety. Even his recollection of childhood is highly sexualized: "...I had three brothers and we bathed with my father until puberty"; however, he does not understand these experiences as sexual abuse, even when I pressed the issue and indicated that such behavior might be seen as sexual abuse in the present historical moment.

Bobby recalls the onset of his sexual life at age 15 when he was able to finally drive and used the family car to frequent a rest stop approximately 20 minutes from his home where he could engage in sexual encounters with men. His recollection of these events is somewhat steeped in shame, which he openly stated during the interview as he recalled his time spent having sex at the rest stop at age 15:

> You know, I was telling John, my fiancé, who's also, who you will also be interviewing, you know that, it's been a while since I really had this conversation out loud about this time in my life and I said it's really—I'm interested to see where I go with—what's going to come out of this because I want to obviously tell the truth but I want now [to] try to tell the story with as little shame language as I can because it was so steeped in shame [Perry: Yeah] for so long. Um, what happened—the bare outline is I became the bell of the ball. I was there all the time, guys knew I would be there. Guys came; I had an attorney from Lafayette, Louisiana, who used to drive over.

Eventually in the conversation, Bobby came to recognize that he was the victim of abuse as a child, despite his own sexual desires:

> Lafayette is about 2 hours and the John Deere dealer, hello, can you get more macho than that, from Pascagoula Mississippi about an hour and

20 minutes. He used to drive over and, I mean to see me, to be a pedophile, you know, to—to—to [be] with me...specifically looking for this 16-year-old. I guess at that point I'd still be—mm? Still a child.

As for many of the men, more than half of Bobby's life is defined, in part, by HIV: "I'm 47, uhh, 24 years. So now I've been HIV-positive longer than—well, more than half my life now as of May of this year [2012]."

Bobby's 55-year-old partner, now husband, John, is more introspective than Bobby. Much of his meaning making is tied to his sobriety from alcohol and other substances, and he often became overwhelmed with emotion as he shared his life events. Use of alcohol and being gay permeate his understanding of HIV and his life overall, as evidenced in this initial description of himself:

Uh, let's see, um, well, I was born in—on Long Island, grew up there most of my life. I think, um, I'm firmly convinced that I—I was born gay, and, uh, and—and born an alcoholic. And, uh, I—I think that the defining moments in my life were figuring out, you know, in second grade or something, that I had these thoughts that made me different from others about men, and then at 15 when I discovered alcohol, and then the—the—the journey from there took a lot of twists and turns, and, uh, um, and I was, you know, it really opened up the alcoholic in me.

John was raised by highly educated and successful parents on the East End of Long Island, his father a physician and his mother an artist, whom he described as "open-minded, liberal, and accepting" and who, according to John, "outed" him as gay "with a great deal of dignity and love and respect" later in his life during his college years. "I come from an amazing family," John recalled.

However, John's experiences within his family were not similar to his life outside of his family, where he was bullied as a child because of his size and because he was perceived as gay. Despite the support of his family, these bullying experiences are informative of how John perceives his place in the world, including his subsequent reliance on alcohol and other drugs:

You know, it—it always amazes me that, uh, and—and it's still—it's—going back to these times is always very painful, and I do it on a regular basis because I speak for Love Heals, so I go to a lot of high schools and colleges and middle schools and tell my story. But, um, and—and a part of it includes talking about what it was like for me being gay in middle school, because they knew, they knew right away.…I mean, no, I wasn't this, you know, flaming little wispy thing. Uh, I don't know how they knew. I—I just—I wasn't into sports or anything, but, um, they knew, and they started, you know, in middle school. When I went from grammar school to the middle school, it included kids from other towns, and it was a group of kids from the next town over who singled me out, and started the bullying, and the "Fem, faggot, gay boy." I didn't even know what those words meant, you know.

These experiences drove John to try to "fit in." John turned to body building, inspired by Charles Atlas, and by age 14 he had grown in size, which enabled him to defend himself from those who victimized him, including the "ring leader" who later in life admitted that he too was gay. The body building was also accompanied by attempts to have girl-friends and sex with women, behavior that led John to his life of alcohol and drugs as a means of coping with a situation that felt unnatural and uncomfortable: "Well, in high school it was—I very rapidly—well, especially after I discovered booze and—and drugs, let's say discovered booze and drugs, I realized that if I was stoned or drunk I could have sex with a woman."

But John's early life experiences, like Bobby's, were also shaped by sexual abuse perpetrated by another man, as well as by his attempts at relationships with women and his use of alcohol and other substances. To date, John believes that he is able to perform with any sexual partner when under the influence, and it becomes clear that the use of substances was initiated by a young man who, although he had the love of his family, was emerging as an adult in a homophobia-laden society, despite the strides made in the 1969 Stonewall Riots that gave rise to the gay rights movement. This is demonstrated clearly in these experiences that were occurring in the early 1970s:

Yeah, and—and that's when I—shortly thereafter, 16 maybe, had sex with a woman, also was having sex with men, I started sex with men early because I was—my—my next-door neighbor was fondling me at 13, and having sex with me, right—and a much older man, and that's how—that's when sex with men started. But, uh, I did, um, was able to, if I was fucked up enough, have sex with women. That—that holds true. Since I'm sober, I've never had sex with a woman, which is why I definitely define myself as gay, but if I'm fucked up enough, I could have sex with anything, you know, basically, anything or anyone.

Richard

I came to know Richard, a 58-year-old actor, pianist, and singer, through my colleague Dr. Antonio (Tony) Urbina, a very well-respected and accomplished HIV physician and researcher, who codirects St. Luke's Roosevelt Spencer Cox Health Center. Richard is a strapping man, over 6 feet tall, with penetrating blue eyes full of enormous wisdom and enormous pain. A son of a Baptist minister who was born in Arkansas and raised in Anaheim, California, and Buna, Texas, Richard's HIV story is one of a pioneer, being the creator of the first AIDS blog, a diary of his life that he developed in the mid-1990s, which were indeed the early days of the Internet. For Richard, many of the critical moments in his life were tied to both his music and his faith, including his first sexual experience with another man:

> When I was 19, I went on a missionary trip to Mexico. I spent the summer in Monterey, Mexico. And I was visiting an older couple. They were missionaries there. You know, to say they're Catholics and turn them into Christians. And uh, on our trip to Mexico City, we went to a larger church, and there was a musician there named Florencio, and he was especially beautiful. And he said, "Oh, I—if you're going to sing, come to my apartment, and I'll play the piano for you." And the minute we got in that room, we were all over each other.

Richard attributes his survival from the ravages of AIDS both to this diary and more importantly to music—the music that he wrote and performed about his disease. It is when he speaks about music that Richard becomes most animated, suggesting the centrality of music to his own identity. Richard describes many aspects of his life, including his emerging adulthood, with regard to music: "And then my education consisted of two years of Baptist college, which is basically a glorified Sunday school with a choir and math. And uh, uh, and then I went on the road as a musician."

Thus, Richard's HIV story is also a story of music. By mid-1994 Richard's health had very much deteriorated to the point that he believed he would soon die, and he describes that period of his life in great detail as he establishes the context for his understanding of how music saved his life:

> I got out of the hospital and couldn't walk, so I had to relearn how to walk just because I was so physically depleted. So I began to rebuild my body one step at a time, one step, back down to sleep. Two steps, sleep for the whole

day. And um, all the people in my office were amazingly supportive. Well, the year before when I told them—when I found out I was HIV-positive, I told everybody in the office immediately. I didn't hide it at all. And uh, got an incredible amount of support from all my friends and the other musicians and everybody else who I knew. Once I landed in the hospital, I had to quit because I physically was unable to work.... So now I'm—I'm spending this year—I was spending this solid year or more doing nothing but trying to build my body back up to, um, some semblance of functionality. I make heavy use of the fax machine. I'm faxing all of my friends. I'm faxing all these people who I knew at NAS, and I'm maintaining massive amounts of communication with everybody who—who I used to know and talk about the progression of the disease and talk about them. And just trying to stay connected to the rest of the world from my hospital bed—I mean, from my—from my home. And spending an inordinate amount of time on the BBS learning about it. And in—and—and also, the other thing I did was, um, when I—when I was either barely functional, I could get up and walk, I would go intern, like an intern for a music agent at one point. And I just sat at his desk, and all I did was just transfer names from here to there. Transfer names from here to here, and just do research work where I could sit at a desk and a computer and just do input because I needed to get up out of the bed and go somewhere and do something.

However, the most significant point of transformation for Richard was the moment he again played music, which is how he understands his entire life, successes, and ultimate survival from near death. Throughout his narrative, Richard refers to the musical he had written, a work he first undertook as a means of combatting the disease and rebuilding his strength in the mid-1990s.

Hal

For 51-year-old Hal, the voice that comes through is that of facing and confronting adversity: "I've always considered myself someone who runs into a fire to save the baby and as far as AIDS and HIV have been concerned I've run to it rather than away from it."

On first meeting, Hal presents as extremely confident. He is strikingly handsome with piercing blue eyes and a well-developed muscular body, traits he uses in a flirtatious manner. This demeanor came across both in our on-on-one discussion and in the focus group. Hal swaggers with confidence as he enters the room; in gay circles he would be described as butch.

However, within moments of speaking and sharing, Hal's emotional and intellectual depth rise to the surface and he becomes much less reliant on his physical prowess, and an incredible tenderness underlies his thoughts, complementing his hypermasculine appearance.

Hal describes himself a "miracle of modern medicine." HIV-positive for at least 28 years, having been hospitalized with his first Kaposi's sarcoma lesion in 1984, and recently married to his high school sweetheart who is HIV-negative, Hal led a young life that was often defined by unsafe sex and the use of substances, all of which radically changed at the time of his diagnosis: "I had a history of substance abuse and when I was diagnosed I stopped doing drugs, drinking. As soon as we knew about transmission I stopped having unsafe sex and began having what, at GMHC, we were calling safer sex." In fact, Hal even applied his talents to the fight against AIDS working at GMHC, the world's oldest AIDS service organization founded by a set of inspiring men including Larry Kramer, who documented the early life of the organization in his play *The Normal Heart* (2000). Hal understands his approach to challenges, including HIV, as genetic:

I come from a family that runs into fires.... They are firemen, nurses, emergency medical technicians.... I was raised to volunteer, to be a Boy Scout.... I have probably normal fears when it comes to everyday life. But when it comes to crisis or stresses I have a very strong lack of fear.

For Hal, like many of the other men with whom I spoke, emergence into adulthood and into sexual life and sexual adventurism was shaped by experiences in childhood with older men. Growing up in Connecticut, Hal describes his first experiences and the onset of his sexual life as follows:

I was in high school. I was in a production of *Jesus Christ Superstar*. The director asked me if I wanted to go to Manhattan. I went to Charlie's on 45th and Eight after seeing a show. The host—there were two hosts and a bunch of waiters. The first host gave me his phone number. The second host gave me his phone number. My waiter gave me his phone number. I asked the guy who—the director who obviously wanted to sleep with me—if he wouldn't mind if I did some exploring. So I went to the first host's house, from there to the second host's house, from there to the waiter's house. I ended up at the Spike and then the Mine Shaft. And then I would go to the Mine Shaft every weekend from then on until it closed pretty much. Got a job as a busboy at Studio 54. Was the most popular kid in my high school. Was screwing Mike [his husband] at the same time I was screwing girls.

Hal's ensuing struggles led to his ultimate confrontation with sex and substance use after his diagnosis, leading to a life of sobriety but ongoing sexual escapism. Throughout the 30 years of his adult life, he continued to have a relationship with his now husband, and within the past 5 years, their ultimate decision to become a couple has shaped his life as he has emerged into middle age. The relationship with his husband also permeates all of Hal's story:

> We reconnected every year for 30 years, two and three times a year, and we would talk about having a relationship and he'd say, "I'm not ready." And I'd say, "Okay." And then I'd say, "I'm ready." And he'd say, "No." Or then he'd say he's ready and I'd say, "No." That went on for 30 years. And then 5 years ago we moved in together finally. We were always with—we were with other people. And we would get together and fuck and our attitude was, "You were my first and I'll never give you up no matter what."

Ryan and Christopher

Ryan and Christopher are the two youngest men I interviewed. Unlike the other men, they both seroconverted just outside the window of the 1980s, in 1991, and the seroconversion came at a time when they both were embarking on new relationships. Both Ryan and Christopher are still with their partners. Interestingly, both also struggle with the source and stories of their seroconversion, which occurred despite each man's belief that he was protecting his health and engaging in safe sex practices. At the time of our discussion, Ryan was 40 years old and Christopher was 45. There is much that bonds these two men, and interestingly I conducted these two interviews back to back.

I had met Ryan some 16 years prior to our interview when we both worked at GMHC and developed a friendship. In 1997, he, with his partner, and I, with my boyfriend at the time, attended the Fleetwood Mac reunion tour *The Dance*. Ryan's relation to me during our interview was indicative of how he views his place in the world, which is often in relation to other people, namely, his family. When I asked Ryan to describe himself, he said, "Let's see. I think Ryan primarily is an activist. Um, starting early on, like in my late teen years. Um, Ryan is very much a son, very much a mama's boy. Um, he's a husband. Um, he's an uncle and a brother. Um, yeah."

Ryan's involvement in activism was defined by both his identity as a gay man and the AIDS crisis, although here these activities are understood in relation to people in his life. Although HIV-negative at the time (1989), Ryan was introduced to and became part of the ACT UP movement through a friend he met at college, who was older than Ryan and whom he was dating at the time. Recalling those days, Ryan describes with great excitement his introduction to Bob Rafsky, one of the leaders of ACT UP in New York City who is featured in David France's documentary *How to Survive a Plague*:

> Um, and he also had a different group of friends that went certainly beyond our college campus. Um, like one night he and I and Bob Rafsky had dinner, um, which like totally blew my mind. Just sitting there, you know, having dinner with him. I didn't realize it at the time. Like, what, how influential he was.

To this day, Ryan is unsure of how he acquired HIV. He recalls the HIV antibody test he undertook shortly after starting to date his now husband as a routine diagnostic during an office visit, not directed by any act that may have put him at risk for HIV infection:

> Um, and, um, I was at my allergist, actually. And I said, "You know what? It's almost 6 months. I should probably have one." I don't know why it occurred to me to say—I think because she was drawing blood anyway. I said, "Could you also do an HIV test?" And she said, "Sure. We can do that." And I said, "Okay."

Being HIV-positive is not the result that Ryan expected. In attempting to identify the source of his infection, Ryan expresses the greatest confusion because of his knowledge regarding HIV at the time and his safe sex practices. For Ryan, this event in his life occurred despite the fact that he postponed sexual intercourse until college and was very knowledgeable with regard to the disease and how it was impacting the lives of gay men:

> Um, it could only have been one of two guys. Um, I used condoms with both of them. Um, I couldn't tell you which one it was because I was seeing both of them at the same, you know, at the same time.

Christopher reminds me of Ryan in many ways, including his physical appearance, that both men are of northern European extraction with fair skin and deep-set powerful eyes, and that both grew up in the New York metropolitan area. Like Ryan, Christopher also seroconverted unexpectedly and during the onset of his relationship with his partner to this day. But unlike Ryan, who was very stoic in his approach to the interview, Christopher engaged in our conversation with a great sense of humor yet still with great introspection. When asked to describe himself, Christopher defined himself as follows:

> It is kind of like a beauty pageant question in that I think for one thing it's always changing. Um, and I—and I—sometimes I think I show the outside world, you know, some people in the outside world something different than, um, I um—that's who I am I think sometimes. Um, it's a difficult question to answer because I'm—I'm kind of always trying to figure out that myself. And, you know the things you wanted at 21 or 22 seem to change—you know, as you get older and, um, I think that, you know, just like with HIV, um, you don't plan that.

Unlike Ryan but similar to many of the other men, Christopher's story of sexual development starts an earlier age while he was still a minor and again with a man who was older, in this case a next-door neighbor, and was focused on foreplay and oral sex. In retrospect, Christopher, 45 at the time of the interview, understands these experiences as abusive and admits that he was even aware of it at the time:

> And I think once or twice we had like sexual experiences, like oral sex or whatever, after that, and I probably, you know, wasn't more than 15, 16. I think I knew in my mind it was inappropriate, but I didn't—I don't think— I think in my—yeah, in my mind I knew it was inappropriate, but I didn't—I didn't really care.

Christopher was raised in New Jersey in a suburban/rural region. His first experience involving anal intercourse was with his high school friend, Raymond, an African American man, who had passed away a year prior to our interview. Christopher recalls this relationship with great affection but also as one of great strain as he grappled with his sexual orientation: "And then I think we were both at odds with ourselves, with each other. I think our relationship for us was a little like living in a mirror. Neither one of us wanted to face the fact that we were gay." More pointedly, it becomes clear that Christopher was very much in love with this man, and it is in this section of our conversation that Christopher is most engaged. It is also clear that this is a relationship that still holds great meaning for Christopher, as he shares how issues of race and class, in addition to grappling with being gay, may have eventually torn them apart. This included Christopher's father's very overt racism. Christopher vividly and with passion recalls his relationship with his lover/friend after high school:

So we kind of went our separate ways after high school. I mean, he was a year behind me so he was there. And he had written me a letter in college and he—he was involved in, not heavy drugs, but he was—a lot of marijuana smoking—while I was still in high school and that sort of just put a rift between us, you know, a further rift between us. And he had written me a letter, I think it was my first semester at college. And I remember reading the letter, going to class and it was snowing out. Like—like—like—and I don't have the letter because I—I was still angry at him. And it was—basically the gist of it was I would rather be someone that smokes pot once or twice a week than be a homosexual like you. He said that to me. And there was a subsequent apology probably a month later in another follow-up letter. And then it was like something out of, you know, Penthouse forum. It was like, you know, like—and it—there was just so much back and forth with him because he never knew where he was or what he was doing.... So I sort of just—I didn't completely close off contact with him, but I didn't make an effort to see him or spend time with him. Like he was a very talented individual, you know, in the arts. Very good vocally and the whole thing. And he wasn't able to afford college. So he wound up, I think, moving to New York and then subsequently Detroit. But there was a moment in there when I had just finished college and I think he was spending his summer up in Provincetown. And I was living with a college friend that summer, so that was 1988. And we—I knew he was out on the Cape, so I don't know how I figured it out, but that was—it was like, you know, an hour and a half for me to go out and see him. And I had a couple days off so he's like, "Come out; we'll spend some time." And the initial 24 hours—well, I had—I saw him for about 2 and a half, 3 days. The initial 24-hour period was like this great, you know, reunion and we saw each other and there was sex involved and all this other stuff. And he lived with a lot of—I don't know how I describe them. I would guess—I would say like liberal, you know, very left-leaning social views and—very progressive and, you know, minority rights and that stuff. And that—these—not all these people were Black or what have you. Um, but there was a point there they all started picking on me because I had like this degree from a very mainstream school in, you know, broadcasting or broadcast management and what was I gonna do for the world? And, you know, I was contributing nothing. And I'm like, "Well, what are you doing?" And like he said, "Well, you know, I sing my protest songs and—." It was like—basically, it was like—you know, and I left there angry and I probably didn't speak to him for the better part of 10 years.

Following this experience, Christopher recalls a series of three relationships that he describes as inappropriate and that in some ways perpetuate the patterns with his first boyfriend because each of the men also struggled with his own sexual orientation.

The striking resemblance to Ryan surfaces in Christopher's recollection of how he found out he was HIV-positive. In this case, Christopher was consistently testing for HIV and was likely detected at the very onset of his infection. He recalls a bout with the measles and an HIV-negative test result at that time, followed by a positive result 6 months later, which he recalls as 1990: "It was—I think I remember watching on the TV that we had invaded the Gulf at that point."

Eddie

Vibrant, intelligent, and effervescent are words that describe Eddie, a 49-year-old African American man. Eddie's journey took him from Detroit, where he was raised as part of a Black middle-class family in a predominantly White neighborhood; to Atlanta, where he briefly studied fashion at Morehouse College; to Newark and New York City, where as a young adult, Eddie found himself unstably housed and homeless. Eddie's mother was nurse and his father worked for Chrysler, and the formative years of Eddie and his brothers situated them for a life of success: "So all our neighbors were White and we were the rich kind of Black, privileged Catholic school kids that are going to go to college and be the fabulous, fabulous people that we know we are." Despite these indicators of success, much of Eddie's life has been defined by great challenges and adversity over and above being HIV-positive. Still, Eddie, at age 49, understands these experiences as key to his identity. When asked to describe himself, he replied as follows: "Um, Eddie, um, Eddie is, um, Eddie stands for something and I represent something. And I like to call it my will, what is wisdom, integrity, and love." And when asked directly about his life's adversities, Eddie indicated,

I thought it was a challenge. I look back now and I think that everything was meant to sort of be the way it was meant to be because that's what made me who I am. I always thought I—when I look at homeless people always, always—I was—at the time, I thought it was the worst scenario I could ever be in. But when I reflect back now, I don't look at it as being sort of a negative sort of down time. I sort of celebrate my homelessness.

Eddie's voice is one of fortitude and savvy as he had to navigate environments and situations to survive, from a very young age. Despite his parents' wishes and hopes for him to become a medical doctor, Eddie went to college to study fashion; moreover, despite the fact that Eddie was raised in the stringent reality of Catholicism and "an extremely disciplined family," he managed to explore his sexuality even at a very young age. Like many of the other men, Eddie knew he was gay as a child, and in his case, he acted upon these thoughts and desires:

I knew something was strange from the age—my first—in first grade. I was 6. It was this little boy who was very curious sexually. And I remember it like it was, I swear to God, yesterday—that he wanted to go into the bathroom with me and we wanted to touch each other. I did. I remember thinking about it at night. I went home and I was thinking about it when I laid in bed. This is what I'm going to do, I'm gonna go in there with him and I'm gonna keep my eyes closed and I'm gonna—you know what I mean? And then I was gonna touch him and then that's it. The next day came, and I went to a private Catholic school. So they had—and the stalls were these real big stalls with—with marble. They were really high and tall. And we were so little that we went into the stall and he leaned on one side of the toilet, I leaned on the other and we were so little that we—that the stall would hide us. And I remember we pulled down our pants and we both touched each other. And someone came in, but we didn't have to do anything because we were little enough so they didn't even see us in the locked stall.

And despite the fact that he was not an alcoholic, Eddie managed to find shelter with the Salvation Army in Newark when he was homeless and in need: "And, um, I love the Salvation Army. It's one of the greatest experiences in my life. I—they took me in. Um, I was not an alcoholic so I pretended to be an alcoholic to get in."

For Eddie, adolescence was filled with sexual adventurism in motels and in the bathrooms of JC Penney, yet, like Gianni, who also was raised in a disciplined, aspirational ethnic family, Eddie hid his sexuality in fear of repercussions and to adhere to societal norms:

I think because, um, everybody else did it, uh, my brothers did it, I didn't understand why I had these feelings, I suppressed them, I wanted to sort of, um, be like everybody else. I did not like the fact that I did that, even though I did. Um, and I used to take my girlfriend out and then after I finished taking her out, come up with some excuse not to really—we only would kiss....I was in high school so I was very responsible, at least my parents thought so. So they would let me have the car and everything because they thought I was dating this wonderful girl who was gonna be my wife.

The voice that reemerged many times during the conversation with Eddie was that of the mentor. Eddie qualifies his role as a mentor by stating that like many young Black gay men, he too struggled with both sexuality and HIV, denying both for many years:

And so I really kept to myself. I had a few, primarily Black, uh, uh, you know, gay friends and we sort of all sort of hung around each other. And um, it was, um, it, in a sense it hit sort of, especially the Black gay community, um, was in super denial about how to deal with this epidemic.

Eddie indicates that the condition is not much improved to this day:

And, and, to be honest with you, they still are. That's the really sad part. That really bothers me, is that there's no sort of excuse. I mean certain communities have done well in general with this disease. And it still is horrendous. And you know young Black gay men, it's horrendous. They still are getting infected and it's crazy. And that bothers me more so than anything else. So, um, and I spend a lot of my time trying to be an example to younger especially Black gay men who just say, "Oh, well, you know! Doesn't matter. I can take a pill; I'll be fine."

Eddie is the embodiment of exuberance. Throughout our conversation, Eddie, who looks youthful and is vibrant and energetic, expressed his thrill at being involved in the book project and grateful to be able to share his story: "And I'm so excited about being in the book; this is like the greatest thing in the world to me. So, and um, life has never ever been better, ever." At the time of the interview, Eddie was in a loving relationship with another HIV-positive man 20 years his junior, which had ended a year later.

Jackson

For some of the men, like Eddie and Gianni, the period after leaving home in the early 1980s for college and other destinations was defined by unabashed and unbound sexual exploration with men, after years of identity suppression to adhere to societal norms. Unfortunately, this was at a time when HIV was circulating wildly in the population, and higher levels of untreated infection led to hundreds of thousands of infections among gay men. For so many gay men, who were promised the sexual liberation of the 1970s, infection with HIV was a situation over which they had no control. This reality was also true for Jackson, a 57-year-old articulate, handsome, well-groomed, and somewhat reserved man, who is the embodiment of Southern charm, and who describes his experience as follows:

> Um, I—I describe myself as a New Yorker. I've lived here since '77, 1977. Uh, I was—I came up here to be a performer, singer, dancer, actor. I grew up in the suburbs of Washington, DC. Uh, and I have a protective realm and got—came to New York as soon as I could, went to college, University of Maryland. And uh, almost immediately—you know, there were 2 or 3 years before the AIDS crisis hit of, you know, the exuberant abandon, and then it all really came crashing down really fast. I was an activist. I threw myself into ACT UP, Broadway Cares. A lot of volunteering.

Born in a family with Southern Baptist roots and strong connections to the church, Jackson was one of five children (in fact, a twin): "So it was a very kind of a conservative upbringing in the liberal pocket outside of Washington, DC." Jackson describes his childhood and adolescence as "coddled," and exposure to drugs and alcohol only occurred during his college years. And like all of the men, Jackson struggled with his sexuality, and this was a source of stress in his life: "I was—I—I—yes. I considered it a happy childhood. I—it was a loving nest. I was terribly closeted. I knew from an early age that—I had the feeling that I had failed my father."

This sense of failure or not living up to expectations permeated much of my conversation with Jackson and seems to have emanated from the perception of how his father viewed him: "I didn't feel uncomfortable. But in the back of my mind, I—I—I—in some dark, mysterious way, I thought I had failed my father. And my father had a temper." However, as an adult, Jackson experienced great support from his parents as a gay man and his perceptions as a child may have been unfounded and informed more by societal norms:

> And then when I came out, my father wrote me a beautiful, supportive, three-page letter full of love and support and would argue far into the night with

my mother saying the gay people…his experience with gay people were hard working, tax paying, respectful to woman, all these values and ideals that he held. And I thought follow more closely in the path of, I wouldn't use the word Christ consciousness, but in the path of Christ; he thought gay people should be exalted by Christians.

As he merged into adulthood as a gay man, first as a bisexual gay man in the mid- to late 1970s ("I loved everybody") and later as a gay man, Jackson struggled with his sexuality, perhaps informed by the religious roots and social contexts of his childhood. In fact, even in this period of sexual liberation, Jackson did not engage in countless anonymous encounters. Instead, he was involved in a series of relationships, the first of which was with his partner Johnny, who eventually died of AIDS:

Well, my first serious relationship, like first lover, was a very intense kind of…actor, singer, director, choreographer who was whip smart, kind of acted up a little probably. And he yanked me kicking and screaming out of the closet. You know, once he realized who I was, he, for instance, would take me to New York, steer me to Christopher Street, grab my hand while we were walking down and not let go, sending me into a blind panic, which by the end of the block was getting kind of like—he said you have to be defiant at first. So I developed, except for my family, a steely sense of sort of being an activist gay.

Jackson's second major life relationship was with another man who also died of AIDS. In fact, Jackson's entire adult life, like that of many of the men, is defined by AIDS: "So now we're—um, yeah. You know, primary relationship. Um, but yeah, as Randy died, Johnny got sick, and one by one, my sexual history, my past, my romantic history was dying off." This reality also is illuminated when he describes first reading about AIDS in *The New York Times*, around 1982, and the loss of his social circle in the years that would follow:

Well, it's interesting because I remember it so clearly reading the article in *The New York Times*. And it happened right over there. One of those penthouses there in an apartment. My friend Dennis had a job cleaning a duplex apartment for a film director who lived in that building. So when the director was out of town, our gang would come up, and we'd smoke pot. It was a perfect arrangement. And hang out. And my friend Martin came in later with the article from *The New York Times*…and, uh, we discussed it. Martin was much more political. Um, he had friends in San Francisco, and he's saying they're talking about this. And then it led to a whole mess into the buzz kill needless to say. And there was a discussion about poppers, and Martin was throwing his poppers away, and Dennis couldn't have an orgasm with poppers. You know, and Martin was our first close friend who died of AIDS, eventually, Dennis also.

And like Gianni, Jackson speaks with a sense of peace about his life currently, married to his husband for 6 years, who referred him to the book project, and living in both Atlanta and New York: "In fact, I'm living—6 months ago, my husband and I moved to Atlanta to be with them. And my husband, works for the CDC, so he was transferred there. So I have an apartment—we have an apartment in New York. We have the best of all possible worlds." Like many New Yorkers, Jackson adds, "…and we're plotting our escape; our return to New York."

Tyronne

Tyronne, a 55-year-old Black man who also has southern roots, came to New York in 1979 as a young man, where a world of possibilities was opened up to him: "Well, I came from Alabama, and I came to New York when I was only 22 years old. I was like an innocent person, living down there all my life, but once I got to New York, and I saw like this whole different world open up to me, all of that went out the window. It was like a whole lot of pent-up stuff inside me just came out." The emotional and sexual release that Tyronne experienced coming to New York City was fueled by a childhood of responsibility and indigence. As a young child, he was removed from school to care for his siblings because of the poverty in which his family was living and because of the large number of children in his single-parent family:

> I came from a very big family. We were very poor, and I mean we always had enough of everything, and my father left my mother with like 10 kids, and I had to spend like 2 years out of school to help take care of some of my smaller siblings, and it kind of made me like an impatient person I think from doing that because I think I so wanted to go to school, and I felt like when my mother took me out of school that it started me to grow in some kind of way, but I mean I just felt stifled, and it kind of made me, because I always held that against her that like she just had something against me, so it kind of made me a mean and impatient person.

Significantly, Tyronne, raised as part of a large and somewhat indigent Black family, understands his acting-out behavior and subsequent behavioral struggles along the lines of these childhood responsibilities:

> I mean one part of it kind of liked it, just taking care of kids. I don't know where that came from. I liked it, but another part was I just felt like it wasn't my responsibility. I mean they were my brothers and sisters, I mean I knew I had to look after them, but I didn't think that I had to take care of them. I just thought it wasn't right for what she did, and I just held it against her for a long time. So then I started growing up, and I started with bailing against her. Everything I wasn't supposed to do, I did. I acted out in school, and then that's when I first started going through the whole thing about being gay. I think I kind of knew it at like 6 or 7, but it was during that time with this thing with my mother where I just said forget it, I don't care. I was tired of hiding it. I started running around with a group of straight guys, you know acting out, to try to prove something. I was in five or six juvenile homes. My mother was like, "You're gonna kill me—my blood pressure." My brothers, my two older brothers before me had been in the same juvenile home, and then I think it was like around 1978, my mother said, "You know, you need to do something."

Compounding these circumstances were Tyronne's same-sex desires and the perceived homophobia evident in his environment:

> I would go fishing. I used to like going fishing with my brothers and his friends, and I have a cousin, he's my first cousin, they used to always play around and call me sissy boy, oh you're not gonna do that, you shouldn't be like this, you need to be a man, blah, blah, blah, come on let me take you fishing. He took me fishing, and he was like, he took his dick out, and of course I was frightened. I so wanted to do it, but still I was frightened. I had heard things about people getting fucked, how it hurts, this, that, and the other because there were like two other guys in the whole town that were gay. Sometimes I would sit on the porch and talk with my mother, and I would overhear them say things. They were like right across the street from me.

And thus it was under these circumstances that Tyronne navigated his way to New York City. In New York, Tyronne reinvented his persona, built his body up at the gym, and worked at the Saint, a very popular and decadent club for gay men in the East Village, which gave rise to the circuit party scene that permeates the gay community to this day. (The Saint closed shortly after the attack of the AIDS epidemic, although it continues to hold events as the Saint-at-Large.) Tyronne embarked upon a series of relationships with three men, mostly White men of Northern European extraction, who became his boyfriends, the first of whom was Jeremy, an English man 20 years his senior who eventually died of AIDS complications, a thought that made Tyronne very emotional. This period of Tyronne's life and the next 20 years were characterized by the continual use of illicit drugs, mostly cocaine, and ongoing short-lived relationships, conditions that existed in his life up until 2007. This time was also characterized by deteriorating health, in part because Tyronne would not adhere to his antiviral treatments because he was selling them to make additional cash to feed his substance use, a practice that was common in his social circle: "That was when people first started selling those things, so I figured well, you know I'm not sick or anything, so I'm not gonna use mine, I might as well sell them like everybody else."

Tyronne also describes this 20-year period of his life as one of caretaking: "I never had anything, so I figured that I could make up for that by trying to fix somebody else...." He attributes his need to care for others to raising his siblings at a very young age, the condition that also prevented him from self-care. However, in 2007, with the onset of middle age, Tyronne shifted the course of his life:

> The fact that I was getting older, and I couldn't keep up anymore, you know, I just couldn't do that physically, and mentally up here. You know everything that I wasn't doing right for my health and myself, it was—I would have to deal with a lot of guilt later. From doing the things I wasn't supposed to do, and then I started to care a little bit more about other people than myself because you know I was kind of selfish you know, I think that had something to do with when my mother took me out of school, I didn't have enough for myself, and I think I tried to get that back later in life.

During the course of our discussion, Tyronne spoke with great enthusiasm about his annual family reunion in Alabama. He has made peace with his family, who has accepted him as a gay man, and in the upcoming weeks Tyronne would be attending this event with his boyfriend, who he has been in a relationship with for 3 years and who is in his early 40s and in need of "fixing," a characteristic that attracts Tyronne to this man in his life.

Patrick

Fifty-one-year-old Patrick, a trained, professional dancer and now a personal trainer, came to New York City from Reno, Nevada. Within the first minute of our conversation, Patrick and I bonded over our admiration for the singer-songwriter Kate Bush (Patrick commented on the albums displayed in my office) and over a mutual acquaintance, whom I had not seen for over a decade. In fact, Patrick indicated that we had met prior to this interview, although I could not recall this meeting. Although these circumstances may have served to facilitate our conversation, in fact, it created a sense of tension that eventually dissipated. Patrick was hesitant at first, either because of our social connections or because of his temperament, but he soon became very clear, articulate, and expressive in his conversation.

Throughout the conversation, Patrick clearly articulated that he did not view himself as a victim, despite a life of AIDS. What comes across is a voice of control and strength, although sprinkled with sadness:

> I've never felt victimized, ever. I've never felt victimized. I've never felt like
> I was going to die. I never felt like I was given a death sentence even though
> I was told that and I saw it in writing.

Patrick describes his formative years as a time of hard work, fun defined by his sexual life and alcohol, and an attraction to older men (his first lover was 7 years older than Patrick), a time during which he moved between Texas, his primary residence, and Oklahoma, Nevada, and New Mexico for his schooling as a dancer and his work as a performer. Patrick believes that his naivety about men and about relationships during this period is the source of his seroconversion. Patrick traces this naivety to the manner in which he was raised, and his story parallels the experiences shared by Gianni with loving yet permissive parents:

> Extremely, very smart parents. Not great at raising a family, children that—
> they were better at making us dismissive and being a family....They raised
> us to be very independent.

Like so many of the men, Patrick's first memories of attraction to men, and again older men, are from a very young age, in this case age 4 or 5: "At the same time, I was fascinated by my next-door neighbor's father." Yet like many of the other men who came of age in the 1970s and 1980s, Patrick suppressed these sexual feelings and desires, even limiting his experiences during adolescence to two men with whom sex was foreplay and attempting to live life as a heterosexual man until age 19:

> And then I tried to have a girlfriend in college. A guy across the hall fixed me up with a girl. There was a girl in the theater department that I was very attracted to, we got along well, and it—I'm sure she knew. Anyway, we attempted to have sex and it was terrible. The cigarette was the best part. And I just knew. And right after that was Christmas vacation. I went home and saw my friends from high school. We went out to a gay bar and that was it.

Throughout the course of his adult life, Patrick faced many of the challenges of living with HIV—the opportunistic infections, including *Pneumocystis* pneumonia and the toxicity of overprescribed AZT, yet the need to earn a living and maintain some semblance of normality. These days, Patrick fully embraces his serostatus, and in fact shares his story of living with HIV/AIDS with his clients, which serves as a source of inspiration to them and a source of liberation for himself:

> I think instinctively now, it wasn't until 2 years ago that I came out to my clients about my HIV status and all the stuff that I'd been through with it. And I started telling one client after another. These are clients that I've had for a long time. Because I, after I told one client who was dealing with breast cancer, that, "You know, I need to tell you something." She's afraid of the doctors, afraid of radiation, afraid of death. I said, "It's okay to be afraid, but you have to—you have to—don't let—you're afraid of the doctor, don't be afraid of the doctor because you have as much right to say 'No' or 'Yes' to anything." And she listened to my little tale about this, you know. And altering. I could see it visually immediately. I helped her. "Wow, really? You've been through that?" "Yeah." "And this is your attitude?" "Yeah, this is my attitude." "And it worked for you?" "Yeah, it worked for me."

Andre

Andre's story is a military story, a life of service to the United States while living with HIV, as well as all the emotional complications associated with these conditions. The story of Andre, who was about to turn 46 at the time of the interview, is a New York City story, a native New Yorker story, which is more rare than one would imagine: "Born in Harlem Hospital. Uh, raised, uh—I have two older sisters. Single-parent household—my mother. Father—well, there was one at one point, but I never lived with him. I really didn't know him."

Andre, a handsome and well-built African American man, was confident, articulate, and extremely intelligent in his presentation and had a smile that lit up my office. Of all the men with whom I spoke, he was the one who most successfully conveyed his thoughts and ideas, because he was very conscious of the structure of his narrative. His story is one of the gifted child, which under the correct circumstances leads to major life accomplishments and in other circumstances, if unharnessed, may lead to the "drama of the gifted child" as described in the profound work by Alice Miller (1997). In this case, it is the story of drama as Andre conveys his acceptance to one of the most prestigious schools in New York City for the intellectually gifted—Hunter College High School—as a situation that was fraught with many issues for him in 1978:

> I get into this school. I'm one of two students who went to the school—we actually made the summer program. One guy was cut from the summer program. I got in and it was really—talk about culture shock. It was, "I don't fit. I don't belong. I can't do this. I can't do this." I didn't have the support. I was the little Black kid for one from down the hill.

The situation was intolerable for Andre, who decided to attend his neighborhood junior high school, and then a public high school, the New York High School of Printing. But for someone of Andre's intelligence (the intellectually gifted child), these environments were not intellectually challenging, and much of his time was spent cutting high school and frequenting the Adonis Theater, a commercial sex environment in the Midtown section of New York City, which was adjacent to Andre's high school. What education Andre did receive in those years was in the form of anonymous sexual encounters at the movie theater: "I would go with my knapsack and check in. And go in there and stay for hours. And I was having sex—oral sex, anal sex, whatever....No condoms, because there was like—who—you know, whatever. What—what's the condoms, then. Right?" Andre's sexual adventurism was not confined to the Adonis and extended into the Rambles of Central Park, the Jewel Theater in the East Village, and the Christopher Street Theaters, environments familiar and iconic to all gay men who came of age during this historical period. (The Rudolph Giuliani mayoral administration in the early 1990s worked diligently to "clean" the city of these sex environments.) In the end, and after a series of trials and tribulations indicative of the drama of the gifted child, including running away from home, Andre easily earned his GED. Andre's first understanding of AIDS as a young man was in these terms:

> It's GRID thing in San Francisco they were talking about. They were beginning to talk about it in New York. And it was the Haitians and it was the gay White man and it was the Haitians and what—"Okay, I'm not either one of those. I'm okay."

Andre's HIV status became a reality during a routine health examination while in the Air Force.

Kerry

My final conversation was with Kerry, a 49-year-old extremely handsome White man with beautiful blue eyes, who likely garnered much attention in his youth because of his appearance and still likely attracts similar attention, despite evidence of some facial wasting due to lipodystrophy. This conversation was joyful as Kerry shared his story after first expressing some uncertainty about the purpose of the interview: "I don't even know what I'm doing, but I'm happy to talk about it." Throughout our conversation, Kerry's smile illuminated the room. I felt very emotionally connected to Kerry immediately because of his sincerity and kindness. This interpersonal prowess also emanated during the focus group when he described himself as follows: "I'm Kerry and I was referred by a friend. And I'm positive since 1992, March of '92 and like everybody else, I'm just thrilled to still be here, I guess."

More often than not, Kerry's voice was one of concern about the realities of HIV, his treatments, his surprise at still being alive, and the effects of the disease on his neurocognitive abilities, of which he spoke quite articulately. His self-definitions were often in relation to HIV. When asked to describe himself, Kerry first said:

> It's difficult, um, and I struggle with it. Um, and I think I've come to terms with the fact that I have to be happy that I'm just here. I still take 26 pills a day. And I—I don't have the energy. And I have—my—my memory's affected by—and, um, it's—it's disheartening in later life in a different way because your family understands—your family and friends understand the immediacy of it in the '80s and the '90s when you're going through med changes and things. But as soon as things kind of level off, they don't realize the repercussions all that has for much later on.

Kerry was the only man who also spoke of the other health conditions that emerged alongside his HIV from years of inflammation (Appay & Sauce, 2007) and also an aging body.

At the time of the interview, Kerry was in a relationship with a man 13 years his junior, who was also HIV-negative, an aspect of his life that Kerry shared with a smile and a sweetness in his voice. When asked about the challenges of being an HIV-serodiscordant couple, Kerry understated the challenge, indicating his limited need for sex (a lifelong condition) as well as the knowledge and confidence he and his partner have with regard to safer sex practices. What becomes apparent is that the relationship is one of mutual support and respect, understanding, and companionship, which was undoubtedly modeled for Kerry by his parents. Growing up on Long Island, New York, Kerry described a loving and supportive family even when he came out of the closet. Of his mother he said,

> She was my buddy. It's a typical gay son, mother relationship. We went to shows together and went to gay bars together and had a great time. Although ironically enough I think she was the one that had a harder time with my homosexuality than my dad. And that was because she wanted grandchildren.

And of his father he said,

> And my dad—my dad sat home and cried one day when he found out that I was gay because he was always the last one to find everything out in the family. But then he was really genuinely more upset that he's always the last one to find out in the family than that I was gay. And my dad invited my lover the first time for Thanksgiving.

But even in this loving family, the reality of larger social circles and society influenced Kerry's development, as it did for so many of us coming of age in this historical period, right after the Stonewall Riots—words that haunt many of us to this day, as Kerry describes:

> I didn't have a gay role model. I remember in, um, I was born in '62, and I have a—there was something that happened—oh, when Harvey Milk was shot. I remember someone in my family saying something derogatory about faggots, and that—I don't remember who it was or where we were or anything like that. And, um, years later I remembered that, but it kind of stuck with me.

Kerry's life journey, however, was also one of struggles—loss of a lover of 8 years to AIDS; a point in his life when his immune system was so suppressed that he had four T cells; a career in the modeling industry that became unraveled because of HIV and the expectation of death, which never came; the challenges of fading memory and the physical complications of entering middle age after an adult life living with HIV; and limited income living in New York City. He expresses a yearning for a time past when he perceived a greater sense of community: "I think the gay community came together in a way in the '80s like it never had before." I expressed a similar sentiment in the foreword for Michael Shernoff's book *Without Condoms* (2005). Michael was a friend and dear colleague and a brilliant psychotherapist who was a pioneer in the development of safe sex practices, a long-term survivor who died of AIDS in 2008 at age 57.

Throughout our interview and in many interactions since that time, Kerry has been articulate, warm, and funny. His kindness radiates through his eyes and his smile. Kerry cites the Broadway actress Megan Hilty, the television show *Smash,* and his dog as his passions. He says, "We make these things to keep us going."

Conclusions

It is the end of July, and the 11:30 a.m. ferry to the Pines on Fire Island, New York, a gay hideaway on the southern shore of Long Island, is more crowded than usual. On this weekend, owners, renters, and visitors flock to the island for the annual ritual known at the Pines Party. This circuit party consists of numerous events lasting throughout the weekend, culminating in the dance party Saturday night into Sunday morning. It is the successor to the Morning Party, an annual fundraiser held by GMHC starting at the onset of the epidemic and continuing into the late 1990s, until the rampant drug use and overdoses and unsafe sex among revelers transformed what was once a somber event to honor those living with and lost to AIDS and to raise funds for a worthwhile organization into a Bacchanalian feast that created a public relations nightmare for the agency. I witnessed this sad situation for GMHC as I was serving as their director of evaluation research at the time. The Morning Party was part of a 20-year tradition of philanthropy and community celebrating on our beach that helped us navigate through the dark hours of AIDS and raise funds for those in need. Since 1999, the Pines Party has raised funds for the Stonewall Community Foundation, which distributes the funds among organizations serving the LGBT community as well as the Fire Island Pines Property Owners Association Charitable Foundation, which enhances the ecosystem and common areas of the Pines. Illicit drug use and unsafe sex still prevail at this event.

On this particular Friday, men of all shapes and sizes merge into a narrow entranceway to board the ferry. Among the 200 or so men ranging in age from their 20s to their 60s are some who are living with HIV, and some who have likely been living with the disease for an extended period of time, like the 15 men you have met. To the normal observer, the fact that some are living with HIV may not seem obvious, but 20 years of conducting this research has sadly empowered me to recognize lipodystrophy (Carr, 2003) (a side effect of HIV antiviral treatment that leads to the redistribution of body fat made most evident by distended bellies and facial wasting resembling Bette Davis in her advanced age). One should never judge or conclude simply from appearances, but in this particular situation, the sign is obvious and clear.

Yet like the 15 men you were introduced to, these men, also in their middle age, went about their business, looking forward to all the weekend had to offer, despite what has been undoubtedly a trying and demanding adult life for them. And like all men of the AIDS Generation, they are alive and a vibrant testament not only to the advances we have made in the fight against HIV but also to the resilience that so many of us have evidenced in the face of a devastating and debilitating disease. I watched these men closely from behind my dark-shaded sunglasses, joyous for their lives but heavy hearted that I could not share each of their stories—but finding solace in my understanding that the life experiences of the 15 men told in the pages that follow no doubt reflect the realities of these men on the ferry—and that like the 15 men in this book, these gay HIV-positive men represent the beauty, strength, and resilience of my generation of gay men, the AIDS Generation.

| Enter HIV

Disease, Diagnosis, and Devastation in the Pre-ART Era

"What should I do?" "What is there to do?" And he [the counselor] basically said, "Well you know, you're a relatively healthy guy, you're in shape. But, but, ya know, I'll be honest with you. You'll be lucky if you live to be 30. So, just go and enjoy your life and, you know, try to say as healthy as possible." And I was like, "Okay. Great." When you are 24 years old you don't expect to hear that you're gonna die in a few years.

THIS IS HOW A 50-year-old White gay man who participated in Project Gold described the story of his diagnosis in 1984.

Prior to 1996 and the development of effective antiretroviral therapy (ART), an AIDS diagnosis or an HIV-positive test result was, quite frankly, a death sentence. In fact, prior to the identification of the virus in the mid-1980s and the development of the antibody tests for detecting the infection shortly thereafter, many gay men became aware they were living with HIV because of the myriad opportunistic infections they were experiencing. And many of these men died shortly after diagnosis of these AIDS-related complications. By 1985, the year in which the antibody test was developed (Pear, 1985), and also the year in which Hollywood screen legend and heartthrob Rock Hudson died, some 1,000 other gay men had been diagnosed with AIDS, and close to another 1,000 succumbed to complications of the disease (Centers for Disease Control and Prevention [CDC], 2012a).

My friend Jim, who was 38 when we first met in 1981, suffered from ongoing sinus infections and cuts that would not heal properly. The glands in his neck and armpits were regularly swollen, and until he was diagnosed with non-Hodgkin's lymphoma in the summer of 1985, he assumed he was just overworked and spent much of his energy trying to combat the fatigue and self-medicate with over-the-counter formulations. By the time of his diagnosis, the cancer had ravaged his body, and within 6 months and without much help from the chemotherapy and radiation he received, he died in January 1986. At the onset of his symptoms years earlier, no one even assumed he had AIDS. But in the last few days of his life, his HIV infection was obviated by the biohazard warning on the door of his Long Island, New York, hospital room and the requirement that we wear surgical gowns, masks, and gloves while visiting him. Jim was an early victim of AIDS, although his medical records and death certificate would never show that.

A major breakthrough in our understanding and management of AIDS came in 1985 when the pathogen that causes the infection was identified and isolated, a scientific discovery fraught with controversy. Both French and American scientists claimed the discovery of the pathogen, known as lymphadenopathy-associated virus (LAV) among Luc Managnier and the French at the Pasteur Institute (Barré-Sinoussi et al., 1983) and human T-lymphotropic virus type III (HTLV-III) among Robert Gallo and the Americans (Popovic, Sarngadharan, Read, & Gallo, 1984). Shortly after a compromise had been reached to share the honor for discovering the pathogen, the AIDS-causing virus was named human immunodeficiency virus (HIV) and antibody testing was developed. To this day, detection of antibodies for HIV consists of two main types of tests—the enzyme-linked immunosorbent assay (ELISA) and the Western blot (WB) (Dewar, Goldstein, & Maldarelli, 2009). In 2012, the oral version of the ELISA was approved for use in home testing (McNeil, 2012), a controversial decision laden with concerns as significant as those early in the epidemic when misuse and abuse of the test abounded (Bayer, Levine, & Wolf, 1986).

HIV antibody testing empowered gay men of the AIDS Generation to learn if they had been infected. But the antibody test also indicated for the first time the extent to which HIV had permeated the gay population. Shilts (1987) depicts this situation while reporting on the San Francisco men's hepatitis B vaccine study (Szmuness, 2005): 1 in 110 blood samples tested positive for antibodies when specimens were drawn in 1978, a number that escalated to 25 of 50 in the specimens drawn in 1980. Within 2 years in this cohort, prevalence increased from less than 1% to 50%, an epidemiological pattern that was being manifested throughout the gay populations in the major metropolitan areas of the United States. It is in this context that the gay men of the AIDS Generation were coming of age, discovering their sexuality, and trying to make their places in the world, and it situated my own first HIV test:

> In 1988, I first tested for HIV. I was 25 years old and had only been out as a gay man for a few years. At the time—which in the history of the HIV/AIDS epidemic was the Dark Ages—my bloods were drawn by my physician, labeled accordingly in the collection tubes, and placed in a brown paper bag. It was then my responsibility to deliver the specimens to the New York City Health Department lab on First Avenue, where I placed the bag through a metal collection chute. I remember this experience vividly, as if it was yesterday, not only because of the fear that numbed my whole body as I walked to the labs, but also because of the rainstorm that had drenched me by the time I arrived at my designated destination. I then waited two weeks for my test results. (Halkitis & Siconolfi, 2010).

In these early days of the epidemic, screening and diagnosis were not differentiable terms. For epidemiologists, screening refers to a strategy to detect a disease when there are no visible signs or symptoms. Even when the test first became available, many gay men who tested were not simply screening for HIV. Many had clear identifiable symptoms; the HIV antibody testing just confirmed what they and their health care providers already knew. This was the case for Olympic diver Greg Louganis. After a bout with a persistent ear infection, Louganis describes being told the results of this test by his physician:

> We started with some informal chit-chat, but I didn't let too much time pass because I wanted to know. I said, "Well what are the results?" He said, "It's positive." And that was it. I nodded my head. I felt strangely calm. (Louganis & Marcus, 1995, p. 177)

All of the men of the AIDS Generation found out through illness or testing that they were living with HIV, and in some cases AIDS, between the period of 1984 and 1993.

Finding Out

There is no simple way to characterize what it feels like to be told you are HIV-positive. To this day this revelation results in a complex emotional reaction, as we have found in our National Institutes of Health–funded cohort study of young gay men (Project 18; P18), where we conduct oral HIV antibody testing at each 6-month assessment. Among those for whom antibodies are detected (i.e., we obtain a preliminary positive result), responses to this news are wide and varied, ranging from extremely calm and silent to inconsolable, from completely surprised to expected, and from embarrassed to unabashed (Halkitis, Barton, & Blachman-Forshay, 2012; Halkitis, Moeller, et al., 2012). However, the overwhelming response is one of shock. Even with our vast medical advances, which theoretically enable those infected to live to a normal life expectancy, the news of a seropositive test result is appalling, even if one knows that he has placed himself in risk's way. I have recently offered to the students in my HIV prevention class a hypothesis that these reactions occur because we are still living in the context and culture of the 1980s when it comes to HIV, a reality also informed by the fact that we still expect gay men to "wear a condom every time" despite clear evidence for close to three decades that this message alone is not highly effective.

Imagine receiving the news during the first decade of AIDS, when clearly and by all indications positive serostatus meant you had only a few years to live. For many of the men I interviewed, that number of years was two. Perhaps this was due to the legend that developed around survival, which I discuss later in this chapter as the "myth of two." For the character Craig Donner in Larry Kramer's play *The Normal Heart* (2000, p. 21), the reaction is combustible: "I'm going to die. That's the bottom line of what she's telling me. I'm so scared."

Put simply, an HIV diagnosis was and is a life-changing event. In 1988, the author and poet Paul Monette documented this experience in the memoir *Borrowed Time*. Monette retells the AIDS story of his partner Roger Horowitz, who was one of the early victims of AIDS and describes how Roger's diagnosis transformed their lives:

> Equally difficult, of course, is knowing where to start. The world around me is defined now by its endings and its closures—the date on the grave that follows the hyphen. Roger Horowitz, my beloved friend, died of AIDS complications on October 2, 1986, nineteen months and ten days after his diagnosis. That is the only real date anymore, casting an ice shadow over the secular holidays lovers mark their calendars by. Until that long night in October, it didn't seem possible that day could surpass the brute equinox of March 12—the day of Roger's diagnosis in 1985, the day we began to live on the moon. (p. 2)

Paul Monette also died of AIDS complications in 1992.

In Project Gold, men spoke abundantly and consistently regarding the often enormous and wide array of emotions that followed after confirmation of status, how this confirmation created a sense of living with a death sentence, and how finding out was a life-altering event. According to one man, "It was a whole bucket of emotions was just running rampant. You know I was angry I was happy I was sad I was ecstatic it was just everything." Another, a 54-year-old Black man, encapsulated these themes as follows:

Um, when I first found out I was positive, um, I was, um, very addicted to ah, crack cocaine, probably about, um, my mid-20s, 26 like that. And um, I was, um, like I said, um, addicted to crack and I was also, um, hustling on the streets in terms of, um, male prostitution. And, um, when I got the diagnosis, uh, it just made me, I dunno, kinda give up on life. You know, so I just smoked and f— myself into oblivion.

And for the Project Gold participant, whose story opened this chapter, finding out he was HIV positive as part of the Multicenter AIDS Cohort Study (MACS; Brookmeyer, Gail, & Polk, 1987) was a reality he did not expect:

When the AIDS started to become an issue, the Pitt Men's study, which is at the University of Pittsburgh, um, was doing this confidential testing just for people just because they wanted to do research. And so for the first couple years they weren't even giving people results because they didn't know what they would tell them actually but I joined the study just for the hell of it; I never thought that I would be HIV positive. I only had one lover since the time it came out and he was the only person I had sex with so I never thought I would end up testing positive. We broke up.

These recollections of HIV testing from Project Gold also align with the stories shared by the men of the AIDS Generation. Most of men of the AIDS Generation cohort came to their lives as HIV-positive men through antibody screening, either alone or with a loved one. For a smaller group of men, diagnosis coincided with the development of an AIDS-defining illness. These stories and the immediate reactions of these men to their diagnoses are examined first; then I examine the "myth of two," and finally I consider the experience of testing positive in an environment where death abounded.

The Pause

During the course of the interviews with the men of the AIDS Generation cohort, one theme emerged more powerfully than any other in retelling their stories of HIV detection. I have come to understand this time after finding out as "the pause," a period of dissociation of the self directly after hearing the news, in which the man is separated from his physical body. This reaction, which was retold in a slightly different manner by each of the men, is rooted in an emotional coping reaction to news that for many of the men was a traumatic event.

What I am referring to as "the pause" is indicative of an acute stress reaction, a diagnosis included in the *Diagnostic and Statistical Manual of Mental Disorders*, fourth edition (DSM-IV; Marshall, Spitzer, & Liebowitz, 1999). Many of the men described this event in their lives as one in which they withdrew from their immediate situations and environments. The immediate result was a numbing and detachment from hearing the news about their seropositivity, a traumatic event each man was experiencing. Koopman, Classen, Cardeña, and Spiegel's (1995) article, "When Disaster Occurs, Acute Stress Disorder May Follow," indicates that this reaction to a traumatic event is a psychological adaptation that mitigates painful thoughts and feelings, which in turn allows the person to continue to function. Physiologically, the acute stress reaction is accompanied by a temporary systemic release of the anti-inflammatory cytokine IL-10 but can be followed by immunodepression (Platzer, Döcke, Volk, & Prösch, 2000).

For many of the men of the AIDS Generation, when news of their status was disclosed, an acute stress reaction ensued as a means of making their way back to their lives, where they could take stock of what had just been disclosed to them and try to make sense of their lives. This reaction allowed each man to manage the immediate situation and is considered a healthy reaction to a traumatizing event, although this ongoing reaction over time is associated with posttraumatic stress disorder (PTSD; Koopman et al., 1995). Previous studies have indicated that this acute reaction may range from 2 to 24 days (see Koopman et al., 1995), and most of the men with whom I spoke indicated that the response was short, sharp, and immediate. Still, failure to manage these reactions over time may explain the elevated levels of PTSD evidenced among HIV-positive men of my generation (Halkitis, Kupprat, et al., 2013).

Michelle Davies also describes this period of first being diagnosed as a crisis stage: "Angst is quite manifest as the individual attempts to adjust to the overwhelming knowledge that death is imminent" (1997, p. 565). She comes to understand this traumatic period as one in which there is a disruption of "lived time" and one's place in the future and one's whole conception of self are likely to undergo radical change (p. 565). This change affects the HIV-positive person's conception of himself, his body, others, and the world around him (Crossley, 1999). Also, according to Reeves, Merriam, and Courtenay (1999), many HIV-positive individuals understand the period between diagnosis and living with HIV as a period of transition, in which they begin to consider how to confront the challenges associated with their diagnoses.

Speaking to this idea of the pause, Christopher, one of the younger men whom I interviewed, described his physiological and emotional reaction when he received his positive test result in October 1991:

> I was very unaware of almost everything around me at that point because I couldn't figure out how it happened and then you sort of go into panic....I guess your heart sort of—sort of sinks into your stomach and you're like, you know, I think because I wasn't expecting it, it just was like, huh? And your first inclination is to panic because you're there alone.

There is no one consistent set of words or one metaphor that the men of the AIDS Generation used to describe the pause, although it was clear that each was speaking about a similar experience with regard to his diagnosis. Each relied on modes of explanation that best captured the physical and emotional aspects in that life-changing moment, encapsulated in the words of Louisiana-born Bobby, who after a series of negative test results seroconverted in May 1988, and describes the moment as follows: "It's deafening quiet and, I mean, deafening loud and completely silent."

At the onset of the epidemic and HIV antibody testing, protocols were haphazard, and until regulations required that pre- and posttesting counseling be provided, results were often released without immediate concern about how such news would affect the person receiving it. Ralph's story is typical of that condition—he was given the results on the telephone while at work in or about 1986, at age 27, while he was living in Utah—and is also illustrative of the disconnection immediately experienced in hearing the news in this medium:

> I worked in a record store back then—actually records. Interesting thing to remember. I remember I was at work, and, um, the doctor had called me and, um, just told me I was—I don't know what they called it. HIV-positive, did they call it that back then? Yeah, it was probably something like that because I don't think it had like a real catchy name to it or whatever. I don't know, but um, I remember I was at work and they—I either called her or she called me, but um, she was matter of fact about the information and I just remember I, um, felt like, you know, the blood flow out of my body. I could feel, you know, all of a sudden coming out of my body. Like, it was a weird experience. I—I felt—if my body was filled with fluid, it all drained like a

sink. Oh, um, I remember I—um, I was at work so I had to keep some kind of, um, sense about me, but um—you know, I just remember that feeling of something draining out of me, um, happening and—I don't know. I never really thought about it, but I never really got it back.

Ralph extended the story and described how that sense of depletion, emptiness, and ultimately loss would only be undone over time: "Like I said, it was like the sink was emptied and then since then to now, the—it's filled up again, I suppose, uh, I don't know, but like I said, it wasn't sudden like that; it dripped into the sink again."

Similarly, the story of Gianni, whose parents had emigrated from Europe and whose home life was steeped in their traditional culture, is also one of physical disconnect and pause when he too was given his diagnosis over the telephone in 1988 at age 25:

> I was at work and had gotten the message at work, and I remember going to a payphone, right, because there were no cell phones, right, and I remember calling the doctor. I don't remember the words that he—I don't even know if he said you were positive. I don't know if you he said, "Oh, you're"—he might have said something like "your results came back positive" or something like that. And I remember just feeling my heart stop beating, and my lungs stopped breathing. And then I packed my bag and went home. I don't remember the rest of that week at all.

Even in 1994, when Kerry first tested HIV-positive and close to a decade after antibody testing was enacted, regulations were still somewhat haphazard. Although attempts were undertaken to deliver results in person, a conversation over the telephone with a health care provider was sufficient evidence to know one was HIV-positive. This depiction is very reminiscent of the story that Kerry, who now struggles with issues of memory, told:

> I was—don't remember how old I was. It was 9—it was 1994. I had gone to the doctor's, like I said for that—then they called me. I actually called them and at the time they couldn't tell you that they were—you were positive over the phone, but they could tell you you were negative over the phone. So I called from my office, which was—I was a commercial, um, an agent for models for commercials. And I just called from my office and said, you know, "Can I get my results?" And she said, "Well, we have to make an appointment for you to come in." And I was taken off guard, but still not floored. And I said, "Oh, well, that can't be good news." And I made an

appointment to go in, and of course I was positive. But I knew from that phone call that I was positive.

Without directly knowing his status, Kerry suspected, took the time to regroup at work and reconcile the information he believed he had just heard, and returned to work. He recalls the images of that period of pause in great detail:

I remember excusing myself to the bathroom—and sitting on the toilet— and staring at—we were at Carnegie Hall Studios and they had those—I'll never forget those tiles that day. They had those like octagonal white— industrial black grout, white octagonal tiles, and then they'd make like deco squares out of them. And I just remember staring at that floor and it taking on all sorts of shapes and spinning and stuff. And then I collected myself and I went back to the office and I turned to the woman I worked with, Cecelia, and I said, "I just tested positive for HIV." And she said—she put her hands up to her face like she was like shocked, and started to cry. And I ended up comforting her. She ended up in my arms crying.

Antoine, who grew up in Brooklyn and first created his life as a gay man in Prospect Park, also retold a telephone story, albeit a somewhat different one. After time in the Coast Guard, Antoine had developed a successful career on Wall Street, where on one occasion in 1985 he participated in a volunteer blood drive. This was the same time that bans on blood donations from gay men were enacted by the Food and Drug Administration (FDA), a policy that despite being highly debated remains in effect to this day (Goldberg & Gates, 2010). Still, in 1985, a year before the FDA ruling, Antoine attempted to donate blood and used this opportunity to find out about his serostatus rather than testing directly with his health care provider. Perhaps this approach eased the anxiety associated with testing, as we have experienced with our research study P18, in which it is clear that young gay men are opting to test with us as part of a study and forego the more sterile and potentially more terror-inducing and impersonal context of a clinic.

Um, I was making my transition from leaving the Coast Guard—and I was working on Wall Street. I was doing like an internship at, um, Irving Trust Bank. And they had a blood drive. And one of my friends who was—we also had a bunch of college together because I did 1 year at Baruch after I left—Bronx Community. I said to her, um, "I'm gonna check this box."

And she said, "Go ahead." And that box was to test to see if I had the virus. And I'll never forget, when I came home, the lady from the blood bank on 61st Street and I believe First or Second Avenue—said, "Mr. Winston, you have to come here because we found some abnormality in your blood work." And I was trying to get her to tell me over the phone, and she was saying, "No, it's against the law. We can't tell—we can't give you this information over the phone. You will have to come in." And so I told my boss, you know—I'll never forget, it was on a Thursday—that I would be there at 10:00 in the morning. And the man came in and said, "You know, we found this virus in you."

While Antoine's response in that moment appears self-assured and confident, in fact it was nothing more than bravado, as is indicated later in our conversation when he describes this version of the pause: "I went, I felt, I went into a cocoon. Because he said to me, 'You basically only have 18 months to live.'"

For Richard, the lifelong musician and composer, the process of testing is one that he avoided until 1993, believing there was nothing he could do if his result indicated he had seroconverted and wanting to avoid the inevitable.

So I thought if I know I have HIV, I'm only going to make myself sick. I'm going to create the disease in my mind. I'm going to make myself sick in my mind. If I can sort of be in half denial, then I'll—I'll stay healthy. But the—because there's no cure for it anyway, so what—what—what matters? What difference does it make?

In truth, the treatment options were limited at that time, and for those that were available such as AZT, the effectiveness was undermined by the toxicity of the drug as well as misinterpretations about appropriate dosing. Thus, much confusion indeed swirled around how and when one should treat with AZT. In the late 1990s it was also determined that a newer drug, 3TC, was highly caustic and could produce life-threatening side effects: lactic acidosis (buildup of acid in the blood) and severe liver problems (AIDSinfo, 2012). Thus, it is within this backdrop that Richard, a highly astute man well versed in the treatment literature, also approached his decision to test for HIV:

I remember making a very firm decision that I was not going to go to a doctor because they didn't have any treatment and thinking, "What—what's the purpose?" And if they start putting me on all these poisons that don't work, it's going to make it worse. It's going to kill me. And—and so I'm just going to—I have—God knows, I probably was infected back in the early '80s....

And despite all the evidence that the test result would be positive, Richard's pause, his reaction to the news, which he describes in great detail, aligns with those of Gianni and Ralph:

> It was a small room. There was a billboard behind, and I think it might have been a straight guy because he had family. Uh, he was a Latino. And uh, he got—I remember him getting my folder. It seemed like time slowed. I remember him opening the folder. And very casually, he said. "Okay, now you have tested positive." And I don't remember anything that happened after that. My mind just went—I was out of my body. All of a sudden, I was thinking of what does this mean? Fuck. I was right. Um, and so I was in a bit of a daze.

And like Gianni, Ralph, Kerry, and Antoine, after this immediate moment of confusion and disequilibrium and within a short period of time, Richard also regained his awareness and made a conscious decision about the next steps in his life, albeit with much more decisiveness about his options for treatment and care, which he had developed through years of immersing himself in the medical and public health literature of the time:

> My reaction to it was to do nothing because there were no medications still that were viable except for AZT and others. And so rather than getting treatment, I left it alone....

Being in a daze, having halted heartbeats and breathing, and being drained are physical manifestations of how many of the AIDS Generation reacted to their HIV diagnoses. Quite simply, the news of being HIV-positive required each man to be outside himself, albeit for a short period of time— a brief hiatus from reality. In this regard, Christopher very intelligently connects this idea of the pause to an acute stress reaction:

> It's sort of like you're very un—I was very unaware of almost everything around me at that point because I couldn't figure out how it happened and then you sort of go into panic. And I remember asking him if I could make a phone call and he said, "No, I can't let you make a phone call here."...I—I don't know if I'd quite describe it like that, but you—yeah, I guess your

heart sort of—sort of sinks into your stomach and you're like, you know, I think because I wasn't expecting it, it just was like, huh? And your first inclination is to panic because you're there alone.

For Patrick, who is a trained dancer and now a fitness instructor, the decision to test while living in Reno, Nevada, in 1987 was driven by news from a former lover who had experienced a heart attack and was at that time diagnosed with HIV. At first Patrick avoided the news, but with the encouragement of a friend who had survived cancer, Patrick decided to test, and he too found out about his seropositive status. And like all of the men's experiences depicted thus far, Patrick also experienced his pause: "Usually when there's news, something like that, there's a pit in the stomach and feel like an intense heat flash." But, like all the others, he too worked through this pause, took stock, and began to plan:

> So, I remember sitting in the car afterwards, sitting behind the wheel with the door open and I was on my way to go to work to do the show that night, and it was like, okay the other shoe fell. And this sucks, but I was thinking about my best friend who had just been diagnosed the year before, and he's just such an incredibly positive, funny, great guy that comes from this little farm town in South or North Carolina. And he just—I thought about him and we had talked about this, the possibility of this happening and so what? You know, this is what it is; you can choose to be funked about it, or look at it this way, you can get hit by a bus tomorrow, so what good would worrying do?

In the case of Andre, an incredibly intelligent and gifted African American man, being diagnosed as HIV-positive had enormous implications that extended beyond his health because he was training as a military flyer. A few days before graduation he learned of his serostatus as part of a routine physical undertaken by the military, which was an early adopter of HIV testing with the establishment of the U.S. Military HIV Research Program in 1986 (MHRP, 2012). A test 6 months earlier had not revealed the presence of antibodies:

> November, I'm called in and I do another blood test. The day before I graduate from my course—my language course—I'm called into the office. And the first sergeant—unit sergeant—sits me down and he tells me that I have HIV. And he said, "HIV." It was—oh, it's HTLV-III. Because I thought, "Oh, maybe I just have cancer or something." . . . And it is—well first off,

you know, there is no confidentiality in the military. The fact that I'm being told by a sergeant versus a doctor or a professional is—and I'm told this and the next question out of his mouth is, "Were you planning on leaving after graduation tomorrow?" "No." "Okay, good." I have to go through graduation rehearsal. You know, we make sure we're going to look good the next day. The commander comes by: "Were you planning on leaving tomorrow?" "No." "Okay, good." Because I am not leaving tomorrow, uh, my—originally I had plans to—I was going to be on flight status.

So for Andre, the need for a pause was even greater because his serostatus had enormous implications for his career in the military and the life he had worked diligently to develop, which he describes as follows:

It was like falling into a hole. I am sitting there and my life, my world—everything's done. Because I don't know what's going to happen at this point. I'm sure they're going to kick me out of—and send me home, but I have to deal with—explain why I'm home.

The Buffer of Love

This feeling of being alone in the period after receiving the news of an HIV-positive result appeared consistently, as is evidenced in the story shared by Andre, in which the news held enormous implications for every aspect of his life, and in the recollection of so many of the AIDS Generation men. For a smaller set of others, the support of a new or existing love relationship empowered them to undergo HIV testing. It is under these circumstances that Jackson, who is the embodiment of Southern charm, and his partner of 8 years decided to be tested:

So we go and get tested. Johnny [his partner] goes in—you know, it was—it was 3 weeks later. At that time, you had to wait 2 to 3 weeks. And actually, it was 2 weeks. But so Johnny goes in first. He comes out and says he's negative. And I go thank God, thankfully for me. And I walked into the counseling room and had to say "I'm sorry, are you saying I'm positive?" because I was so sure we were the same thing. And it threw me into just the illogic of it. The facts just didn't make sense that we would be serodiscordant just—because I like to figure things out. I like there to be a reason. There was no reason.

And even with Johnny right next to him, Jackson experienced that moment of learning about his disease—the pause: "But and unfortunately, as close as we were [referring to Johnny], you know, also sitting in that chair next to him, I felt like I was on a different planet. I felt so far away from him." In fact, this period lasted for much of 6 months, during which Jackson shut off his emotions:

> I shut down emotionally, which is generally the way I deal with, you know, shocking news, you know. I—she was saying do you understand what the test—yes. I didn't cry for 6 months. I didn't cry—the reason I cried was I had gum surgery where I was in such agony from the gum surgery and the drugs. Then when I released it all, it was—I cried buckets. It was like howling. I had to put a pillow over my mouth because I was afraid someone would think someone was being murdered.

For others, as is the case to this day, testing is undertaken upon entering a new relationship. In the literature this phenomenon has been explained as an attempt to make sure that both members of the dyad are healthy, to negotiate their condom use, and to determine the rules that govern sex within the relationship. These are the tenets that direct a current initiative targeting gay men in the United States known as *Testing Together.* This work is directed by a broad range of behavioral research providing support for the idea that gay men often seroconvert in the context of main relationships (Hoff et al., 2009; Sullivan, Salazar, Buchbinder, & Sanchez, 2009). Such couples-based HIV testing and counseling has been shown to be highly acceptable by gay men (Stephenson et al., 2011).

Of course, the science of couples-based testing has emerged 30 years into the epidemic. In the 1980s no such behavioral research was directing the actions of gay men. It was their gut instincts that drove them to test for HIV in the context of the relationship. The science has finally caught up to the practice, as has so often been the case in the field of HIV prevention, where the best work is conducted on the hyphen of theory and practice.

I also believe that a new and emerging relationship provides a buffer against what may be a life-altering event. Although the news of a positive result nowadays may not have the same dire consequences today that it did in the 1980s, it is conceivable that for a young man emerging into adulthood, the process of falling in love can provide the power to take control of his own health, and that testing in such conditions aligns with the ideas of the behavioral research but also transcends simple behavior and taps into human spirit, kinship, and strategies for survival.

Among the men of the AIDS Generation, both Gianni and Tyronne recount their experiences of testing vis-à-vis their new relationships. For

Gianni, these associations are very clear as he describes his emotions in 1988 upon first meeting his partner and first great love, and the power this developing love provided for him to undertake his first HIV test:

> People are starting to figure out that...it was not until 1985 that the virus gets identified and antibody test in 1986 becomes readily available in 1987. People are talking about it, there's movements afoot, but it's not like, um, for me, personally, at that point as a person who is not really involved in a big gay circle that there was like death all around me. No, there was not that. I didn't see any of that until later. And then everything changes when I meet David [his partner] in '88. My world dramatically changes. I test—I meet David—I meet David at the Eagle, um, wearing this little white T-shirt and jeans, and we walk to his apartment, which is on 13th Street....I can see this so clearly in my mind. I remember getting closer to the apartment and David saying to me "Well, I just wanna tell you that I'm positive," and I said to him "Well, I probably am too." Um, and then—'cause I was pretty sure I was....So it's March I met him, March 26th, can't rem—, remember these dates, I wanna say like May I decide that I should test....I'm okay because David has given me strength somehow to do this. I'm in love; it's like it's all okay.

In a similar vein, Tyronne, who came to New York in 1979 and worked at the Saint, recounts how he and his new boyfriend decided to test together in 1988. Although they did not undergo testing side by side or on the same day, they both tested in the context of their new love:

> I heard, I heard a little something, I think like I heard something, but it wasn't until like I think like '86 when I really, really—I was with someone else then. I was with an Irish kid then. He was like younger than me. His name was Mikey. He was a good guy. He was a very good guy, and it's just that I figured that we was gonna be together forever, and I was like, "You know, I think we really need to go and get tested." I was like, "You go get tested first."

And for Tyronne and his lover at that time, the testing process was not driven by an abundance of behavioral research. Instead, their instincts directed their actions, and their test results within this context provided them each with the support to handle the news:

> I said, "Well what will you do if you test positive?" He was like, "Well, I guess I'll deal with it." I was like, "All right, and I promise you that when

you come back, I'll go." So he told me—and it was like—[he was positive] and I was like, "Damn." I was like—the first thing I—it was like, "Look, I didn't give it to you." You know, he was like, "I didn't say you gave it to me." He was like, "Why don't you go and get tested, you know, and let's see what's up with you." I went there like 2 weeks later. And I was positive, and when they told me, I was like, "Damn."

Then, like so many men, Tyronne described the pause followed by a clear course of action to take:

For like 5 minutes I felt really depressed, and really sad, and after that I was like—the lady was like, "Are you okay?" and I was like, "Yeah, I kind of expected it anyway."...We made this pact then—whatever happened, we would both die together because we were lovers for that while, and that no matter what, we were gonna be there for each other, and if we had to do the suicide thing together, that's what we would do, together.

For John, Bobby's current partner, testing was embedded in a loving celebration, Valentine's Day, with his partner at that time, Peter. His test result was also delivered on a special week of his life, his 30th birthday, and his annual St. Patrick's Day celebration.

And Peter and I got back together. And, um, in 1987, for Valentine's Day, he said, "My gift to you is, um, I got us a test in Chelsea, in a clinic to go get tested for the—for HIV."...But we went, uh, Valentine's Day of 1987. We went to the clinic. They—they took the blood, and then we had to come back 2 weeks later. Well, March 15th of 1987 I was turning 30, and my parents were—my brother, and my parents, my family were having a big party out in, um, Westhampton. And Westhampton has a St. Patrick's Day parade. That year—it—it's always the Saturday before the 17th. So that year it was on the 15th, which is my birthday, and my brother was doing a float in the parade, and I was gonna be on the float as a mermaid. I did that for many years. And that's all I could think about, was I was so excited about this whole thing. And—and not that I'm big into drag, but it was such a hoot, you know, to do that in my hometown. And, um, we went back for the results. And he went in, and he was negative. And I went in, and I was thinking about, you know, my costume, and how many people were gonna come to the party, and—and she said, "You're HIV positive." I never even expected it.

How Did I Get Here?

As is evidenced in John's recollection of HIV testing, news of a positive test result is one that he had not expected. Across the stories of the men of the AIDS Generation, three types of understandings of this life-altering diagnosis emerged. Like John, who continues to live on Long Island, there are those for whom the news came as a surprise and was not a situation they had fully foreseen. Within this group there are two types of men: (1) those who had no clear evidence in their lives based on their behaviors that they should be HIV-positive, who I will refer to as "the unexpected positives"; and (2) those who, like John, and despite the evidence in their lives, continued to believe that they somehow had escaped infection, who I will refer to as "the avoidant positives." However, the voices that most often appeared in the stories were those of a third group—a group that experienced little surprise at the time of diagnosis, "the expected positives."

There is no doubt that many of the men of the AIDS Generation had expected the news they were to receive when first testing for HIV—the expected positives. For these men, there was also an underlying belief that they were likely to be infected based on the experiences in their social and sexual circles and based on their own behaviors. This is the mindset with which Richard, whose music helped him through the darkest hours of AIDS, approached HIV testing in 1993, and also is clearly evidenced in the recollection of Gianni, who said,

> I knew I had to be positive. There is no way I could not be. I just didn't want it to be real. It's like a little phone and I call this guy and he tells me over the phone that I'm positive. And I didn't fall apart, I didn't. I expected it.

Antoine, who lost almost his entire friendship circle to AIDS, also was not surprised. Recalling his interaction with the counselor at the blood bank, Antoine described his reaction as follows:

> [The counselor asks,] "How do you feel about this?" And he was in shock because I said to him, "I've been in every bath house from here to San Francisco. It would be a miracle for me not to be positive."

In the case of Bobby, now a school teacher, his sexual adventurism throughout his adolescence and early adulthood led him to believe that he was living with HIV. In fact, he describes continually testing at his local department of health, knowing that at some point the results would be positive, as reflected in his retelling of that event and the word uttered by the social worker who delivered the news:

> She said, "Well Mr. O'Hara, I see that, um, you have been tested with us before. I see," she said, "well it appears to me you kept coming back until you got the answer that you wanted." And she wasn't being cruel.

For a smaller set of the men, there was a sense that somehow they had defeated the virus and avoided contracting the disease. These I have come to know as the "avoidant positives." In the 1980s, Jackson, who was very involved with ACT UP at its height in New York City between 1988 and 1993, was experiencing great loss in his life. By 1989, the year in which he tested for HIV, one by one former lovers and members of his theater community had succumbed to AIDS. In this same period, Jackson was deeply immersed in the AIDS activist world and the literature, and despite all indicators from his sexual history, Jackson had convinced himself he was not ill, in part reconciling this evidence with the fact that he had been in a monogamous relationship during the prior 8 years. Although two of his former lovers had died in this time period, they were lovers from the early to mid-1970s, and in the midst of the ongoing barrage of information and misinformation we were all experiencing, it is conceivable that one could come to the same conclusion as Jackson about his serostatus. This uncertainty about whether one could be infected is attributable to stories such as this that appeared in *The New York Times* on June 18, 1982 (p. B8):

> Scientists are using "as many ways as we can think of to identify" the infectious agent in the laboratory, he said. However, the epidemiologists said in their weekly report that they were still considering alternative hypotheses. One, they said, is that sexual contact with patients with GRID syndrome does not lead directly to the breakdown of the immunological system, "but simply indicates a certain style of life. "The number of homosexually active males who share this life style," he said, "may be much smaller than the number of homosexual males in the general population." Still another hypothesis under investigation is that the syndrome is related in some way to drugs, other environmental agents or some other common factors not yet detected.

This article by Lawrence Altman (1982b) was indicative of our understandings at that historical moment and for much of the first decade of the epidemic. (I was recently reminded of the power of Altman's writing in our lives as I again watched the harrowing film *Longtime Companion*, the opening scene of which focuses on the central characters reading these first accounts of AIDS.) Maybe some of us who were not widely sexually active, who were not using drugs, and who had avoided bath houses had been spared. In hindsight, our thinking, of course, now seems odd and flawed. But we were all grappling with this challenge, witnessing the devastation AIDS was causing in our social circles, and none of us wanted to die at the prime of our lives. It was not until Martin Delaney, a very well-respected activist, encouraged testing in 1989 at a meeting of ACT UP in New York City that Jackson finally took the steps necessary to determine his serostatus. In this case, the messenger's message was highly effective:

> So in 1989, Martin Delaney came from Project Inform, and here was this guy in a V-neck sweater, which looked warm. And you know, not looking like an ACT UP person. But he looked and sounded very rational and normal, which is like a drop of rain in the desert....So we went to the teach-in, and he laid it all out, you know, logically. He says you want to—finding out whether you're healthy, you can make decisions. You can change your lifestyle, and you can buy yourself a year or two, which could make all the difference.

Among the men of the AIDS Generation, there were two men with whom I spoke who were neither expected positives nor avoidant positives, but unexpected positives—the men who had no viable evidence that would lead them to believe they had seroconverted. For Ryan, whom I first met working at GMHC, the news of an HIV-positive diagnosis was much less expected than for any of the other men with whom I spoke. To that point in his life, Ryan had only had sex with two men, used condoms for anal penetration, and was highly knowledgeable about the disease given his involvement in ACT UP. Moreover, the HIV test that he undertook in the fall of 1991 was part of his health-seeking behavior, which had greater significance as he had just initiated a new relationship with his husband to this day. Yet like many of the other men, even those who suspected a diagnosis would be confirmed, for Ryan, the period immediately after the news was characterized by a similar immediate emotional and physical disconnection and reaction:

> Um, so I went to my doctor's office, which was the allergist, only like three blocks away. Um, she told me that it came back positive. I was completely

in shock. Um, I walked back home in complete silence. Um, got home, threw up, um, sat there for a while, and then called my mother.

At around the same time in 1991, and only miles away from Ryan, Christopher's story of being diagnosed emerged in a very similar way. Like Ryan, 49-year-old Christopher, who had been very careful in his sex life, had routinely been tested and had no convincing evidence in his mind as to why he should receive a positive diagnosis, and he too had just embarked on a new relationship with his partner to this day, Bruce:

> It was October 3, 1991, and I remember thinking it would be pretty easy because, you know, I had—I think I had gone there—I don't think it was a year prior. I think that was 2 years prior to that because I had had the one test, then I had the test at the hospital, and then I had this one. So I was expecting a negative result—because there was no reason to believe that I had it.

For both Ryan and Christopher, there was little preparation for the news they heard from their health care providers. Unlike the expected and avoidant positives, who possessed a core sense, consciously or not, that they were living with HIV, neither of these men approached their seroconversion with this foresight. For those who expected the result, there had been time to prepare, to rehearse the scene for the possible outcomes. In the case of Ryan and Christopher, the news was shocking and unexpected, much like the terrorist attacks on 9/11, but much more personal and without the camaraderie and support of an entire grieving country. There was no time to prepare and, as we all did on 9/11, to quickly gather our thoughts, remain calm, and develop a course of action. Christopher recalls the events of the day after a series of negative test results throughout the prior year and no sexual behavior that could be considered high risk:

> And I remember him [the clinic worker] telling me and I flipped out. Like I didn't like go crazy, but I was just like...I mean, you know, you go back and, um, like at the end of—all—all of a sudden like the world just goes away and you're like—it's sort of like you're very un—I was very unaware of almost everything around me at that point because I couldn't figure out how it happened and then you sort of go into panic. And I remember asking him if I could make a phone call....

No Time for the Pause

In the stories I have retold thus far, detection of HIV infection was determined through antibody screening. But in the 1980s it was not uncommon for gay men not to be diagnosed with AIDS until their disease had rapidly progressed, as was the case with my friend Jim or as shown in the stories shared by Michael Callen (1990) or depicted in the film *Longtime Companion*, where several of the characters became aware of their condition only when they develop an opportunistic infection such as *Pneumocystis* pneumonia or Kaposi's sarcoma. Describing early victim Ken Horne who was being treated at St. Francis Hospital in 1981, Randy Shilts (1987, p. 59) describes this situation:

> Ken had been suffering from unrelenting fevers for weeks now and complained of increasingly severe headaches, and today that pounding pain. Ken had become testier with each passing month. He didn't want any more tests; he just wanted to know what he had. Meanwhile he deteriorated. New lesions appeared on his face and palate in February. In early March they began covering his lower back.

For so many gay men in the first few years of AIDS who learned of their conditions through the complex diseases they had developed, there was little time for a pause as their diagnoses occurred within the context of AIDS-related complications that were compromising their lives. Some were afflicted very early in the epidemic (i.e., prior to 1985) when monitoring for HIV disease was neither routine nor standard, whereas others simply avoided confronting the possibility of HIV even after the advances of antibody testing and initial treatment in the form of AZT had emerged as a potentially viable treatment in 1986 (Fischl et al., 1987; Levine, 1986).

Among the men of the AIDS Generation cohort, this was the case for Connecticut-born Hal, who returned to his hometown as he grew progressively more ill with night sweats, lymphadenopathy, and a low T-cell count, and who describes first finding out about his AIDS diagnosis as follows:

> I was in a hospital in 1984 in Norwalk, Connecticut. I was the only case. I was in an abandoned part of the ward. I was by myself with signs on my door saying "Hazard." I had to take my Band-Aid from blood tests off, put it in a plastic bag, close it up, put a hazard sticker on it, put it in the trash bag, close that up, and put a hazard sticker on the trash bag. And at 9:00 on

November 21, in the morning—in 1984, a doctor came in and said, "We think you have this new gay disease."

Yet even after this devastating diagnosis and serious bout with complications, Hal, like many of the men, took charge of his life, in this case turning to one of the few venues where he could be with others experiencing the same life-altering events: "So I came back to New York to 18th Street and joined the Gay Men's Health Crisis."

The story of Eddie, who was raised in a middle-class Black family in Detroit, is also one of simultaneous illness and diagnosis with AIDS. After a brief time in Atlanta, he dropped out of college and returned home to Detroit, where odd jobs supported him until his body weakened. When asked about how he was first diagnosed, Eddie struggled to recall these events in his life in 1992. At this point, the HIV antibody test had been available for at least 6 years, and Eddie had been diagnosed with a series of sexually transmitted infections, a condition that should have been a trigger for testing. Still, Eddie, did not test until he experienced illness and was hospitalized:

EDDIE: Gosh, it's so much. Um, I remember getting sick. I was working and, um, I got—

PERRY: Working—working as what?

EDDIE: This was in Detroit when I—when I didn't finish college and I went back home and so I was working and I was doing, um, I just—this voice of mine, so I was doing sort of call—telephone work.

PERRY: Telephone work, got you.

EDDIE: Yeah, and I got violently sick. I had to go to the hospital.

PERRY: Well, how sick? What—what did it feel like?

EDDIE: Fever.

PERRY: Got it.

EDDIE: Nausea, diarrhea, I think. Just—

PERRY: Where are we? What year is this?

EDDIE: 1992.

PERRY: 1992.

Death Sentence and the Myth of Two

To this day and even with the advances in the treatment of the disease, an HIV diagnosis is still a life-altering event. But in the period before the implementation of effective antiviral therapies, the consequences of a diagnosis were even more profound. As early as 1990, it was apparent that AZT (aka zidovudine and azidothymidine), first available in 1987, was toxic (Richman et al., 1987) and did not bestow the benefits needed to combat the virus (Hazuda & Kuo, 1997). As the 1990s emerged, AIDS cases among gay men continued to exponentially grow, peaking between 1992 and 1993, and deaths continued to occur, reaching their highest point for gay men in 1994 (CDC, 2001).

In fact, 1994 was bleakest, darkest, and most deadly year of AIDS in the gay population. That is not to say that gay men are no longer dying. In fact, in 2009, there were 6,863 such deaths (CDC, 2012b). But the outlook was much more grim prior to 1996, as captured in the words of Greg Louganis, who was interviewed by Piers Morgan during the 2012 Olympics (CNN 2012): "Back in 1988 when I was diagnosed with HIV, we thought of HIV as a death sentence." Louganis proceeded to say that he did not believe that he would survive to age 30, a sentiment expressed by many of the men with whom I spoke, including Antoine: "[I had to] stop thinking that I had a future. Stop thinking that I was going to make it to 30."

This sense of life ending within a brief period of time expressed by Louganis was the sentiment almost all of the men of the AIDS Generation experienced and expressed. This notion that time was limited resulted from what these men had witnessed occurring in their own social circles, what they had read, and what they had been told from others, including those in health care. Explaining why he went into a cocoon upon hearing the news of his HIV status, Antoine recalled the words of the blood bank employee: "Because he said to me, 'You basically only have 18 months to live.'" This was despite the fact that Antoine had no visible symptoms or infections; this information or misinformation on the part of the testing counselor ultimately altered the path of Antoine's life:

> And did I pay for his being wrong. Because in those 18 months, I figured, well since I only have 18 months to live, let me max out all of my credit cards. Let me just go wild and reckless. And it was 40 of us that had made a pact.

Similarly, upon receiving the news of his status, John, who married Bobby months after our initial meeting, also was convinced of his imminent death, which was informed by his own experiences to that point in the epidemic and the contradictory yet obvious message being given by the testing counselor:

> And she said, "You're HIV positive." I never even expected it. And I think I—I almost passed out. Because in 19—you know what it meant in 1987.

It means pack your bags, you're gonna die. Any day. And I started—and I looked at her, and I—I must have turned white. And she said, the only counseling I ever got, "Honey, try not to think of it as a death sentence. You probably have a year to a year and a half before you get sick." And—and I looked at her, my eyes went like this, and was—what I was feeling was, "don't say die." And she left it out, very kindly, "get sick," and she said, "So good luck." And that was it.

And for Ryan, my Fleetwood Mac–loving friend from GMHC, the unexpected news of a positive result, followed by the pause, then gave rise to this set of thoughts:

Oh, I immediately pictured my grandparents and my parents at my funeral. I mean, this is 1991. I immediately thought, you know, "I'm gonna die soon." I mean, that's—there was just no question about it. Um, I mean I don't remember a specific number, but I do remember, you know—I remember envisioning my grandparents at my funeral, so that meant it wasn't too far off. Because they were old.

Patrick, who was shuttling between Nevada and Texas during his dancing career, was not convinced of his imminent death, but his friends were less hopeful. And in 1997, despite recent medical breakthroughs, those around him were witnessing a deterioration and believed that Patrick's demise was sure to follow:

After that I didn't think I would ever perform again. This one theater company I had worked with several times actually gave me a dinner, a dinner in my honor because I'd worked for them so much. Totally not—clueless about it—I just thought it was a dinner because they appreciated me. They thought I was going to die. I said, "What?" "Yeah we were all kind of—we just wanted to know that you had support and blah, blah, blah. And very afraid that you were going to die." That's what that dinner was about?! Really? So, I had no clue.

For handsome, blue-eyed Kerry, whose flourishing career was derailed by AIDS, the notion of his mortality was informed by watching his former lover's friends succumb to dementia: "I'd just seen...two friends literally go crazy in a room and die." This was also the case for Hal, who, in 1984, had been diagnosed with AIDS in the Connecticut Hospital and then proceeded to GMHC, where he witnessed the havoc AIDS was creating:

> PERRY: So the doctor in Connecticut comes and tells you probably have this gay disease, this GRID thing, and I think we're probably still calling it GRID at that point.
> HAL: Yeah.
> PERRY: And what's your reaction?
> HAL: I'm gonna die.
> PERRY: And how quickly are you gonna die?
> HAL: Like tomorrow. It was pretty—I've always had really horrible death anxiety about—and I think it was—it got a lot worse working at GMHC and seeing so many guys with KS on their face or cytomegalovirus or PML or any of the diseases, watching them die these horrible, horrible deaths. I just assumed I was next. And I had an HIV doctor at Beth Israel that said, "I would give you 2 years."

This notion of 2 years was also what the health care providers in Detroit indicated to Eddie in 1992: "I don't feel like I'm sick but I've got this disease and they told me probably I would live a couple years." And for Andre, who found out during his military training in or around 1986, the diagnosis left him with enormous fear of the inevitable:

> Uh, I'm going to die within 2 years. I got 2 or 3 years, tops. Maybe I should kill myself because, uh—it's gonna be an ugly death, you know? You've seen—I've seen the pictures. You know, people get thin. They waste away. They die. Like I don't want to do that. That's gonna be painful. Why don't I just kill myself, you know?

The diagnosis led to many strategies for survival. As we will learn in Chapter 4, one of those strategies was an attempt to escape through the use of alcohol, other substances, and sex. For Bobby, this was the immediate recourse until he could reconcile his emotional state, which he described in the focus group as follows:

> I think the first thing I did—and I'm only a little bit joking, is to completely go into denial. After the first 2 weeks of sobbing my eyes out, fiddle dee dee. You know? I couldn't spend every waking day, every waking moment of the day thinking, "Ah, I'm gonna die in 2 years." So I didn't. And I began

perfecting my drinking problem, which continued on for years—so at first, run—running away from it was the only way I could live with it.

Given our understanding of the disease in the first decade, it is clear why the "myth of two" emerged. This is depicted in the opening paragraph (p. 1) of Michael Callen's 1990 work *Surviving AIDS*:

> I was diagnosed with AIDS before the term AIDS even existed. It's been nearly eight years since the doctor told me I had what was known as GRID—Gay related Immune Deficiency.
>
> According to the best estimate of the 1,049 Americans diagnosed with AIDS during 1982, twenty-five are still alive.
>
> I am one of the lucky ones.

These life expectancies are in sharp contrast to where we are in terms of treating and maintaining the disease today. According to the Antiretroviral Therapy Cohort Collaboration (2008), nowadays a 20-year-old who is detected and treated may live to age 69 if he adheres to treatment and maintains a healthy lifestyle. Not only is this an improvement in the days before antiretroviral therapy (ART), but also it represents a 37% increase in life expectancy from the early days of combination treatment (i.e., the late 1990s). Furthermore, this is in sharp contrast to what Callen concluded in 1990 (p. 22):

> Without knowing much about statistics, I decided to define long-term as anyone who has survived twice the current median survival time. In 1987, the median survival time for a gay man with KS was about eighteen months, so I chose thirty-six months (three years) as my arbitrary qualifying point.

This definition, in effect, led Callen (p. 26) to the following point: "And so after a long, convoluted journey through a jungle of conflicting statistics, I have confirmed that one in ten of us diagnosed in the early days have earned the term long-term survivor."

This is all to say that the "myth of two" was, in part, accurate and based on evidence. In the very early days of the epidemic, people were diagnosed with infection and experienced high mortality rates. In fact, even the behavioral academic literature portrays anyone living beyond a few years with a diagnosis as a long-term survivor. Barroso (1997) defines long-term survival as 3 years; Davies (1997) defines long-term survivor as anyone living with a diagnosis for 5 years or more. However, in these early days marked by confusion, those with very progressed disease who were diagnosed with clinical manifestations (i.e., full-blown AIDS as defined by the CDC [1992]) were grouped with those who simply tested seropositive and had no visible signs or symptoms of disease or any of the CDC-defined markers of an AIDS diagnosis. In other words, anyone with any form of diagnosis, be it positive antibodies or advanced opportunistic infection, was grouped together. This may not have been the scientific understanding, but it certainly was what those like the "average gay Joe" likely believed. For the reader for whom the terms "AIDS" and "HIV" are synonymous, I provide a point of clarification. One can be infected with HIV and be HIV positive and not be diagnosed with AIDS. One becomes diagnosed with AIDS after a bout with one of the CDC-defined infections or when one's blood markers, specifically CD4/T-cell counts, reach a low threshold (200 per microliter) as per the 1993 case definitions. In 1999, the CDC also established case guidelines for HIV infection to distinguish this condition from full-blown AIDS.

What we know now is that HIV disease progresses over time: first infection, then AIDS-related complex (ARC), and then AIDS (Weeks & Alcamo, 2010, pp. 94–115). Those with clinical symptoms in the form of opportunistic infections have AIDS and were infected at much earlier points in their lives. In effect, a gay man presenting with Kaposi's sarcoma (KS) in 1982 would likely have been infected years before, possibly even a decade before, the development of KS lesions, because most health models suggest that untreated AIDS will develop within a decade of infection (Fauci, Pantaleo, Stanley, & Weisman, 1996). Osmond (2008) showed that 51.2% of gay men would develop full-blown AIDS 10 years after seroconversion, and less than 1% within the first 2 years, providing further support for the ideas presented here.

Still, for the men of the AIDS Generation, such information was not always clear and apparent. And as we know from the world of research, the translation of knowledge is often slow and in some cases absent. What we, all gay men, positive or negative, saw during these dark and painful years was friends dying around us and portrayals in films like *Longtime Companion* and *Philadelphia*, where men quickly perished and suffered painful deaths. There was no reason to believe that the "myth of two" was incorrect. And so the men of the AIDS Generation bided their time and waited, hoping, as Jackson describes, that an effective treatment would be developed:

> Well, and I thought of it in terms of I will need another year, I need an extra 2 years. You know, if I can get through 2 years, maybe there will be another medication, you know. And you know, I was lucky I guess.

This breakthrough would not arrive until 1995–1996 and after so many of my generation had lost their battles to this disease. In the interim, many of the men simply lived through the pain and horror, expressed in the words of Tyronne upon learning of his diagnosis and returning home to his partner:

> Yup, I was like oh my God, I do not want this slow agonizing death. Am I gonna try to do this in private or what am I gonna—I'm not gonna commit suicide, that's what I was thinking, and I got back home, and I told him.…

For some of the men, like Kerry and Ryan, this understanding of imminent death changed the course of their lives and led them to decisions that have repercussions to this day. Kerry abandoned his successful career and now struggles with how to kick-start his life again, and Ryan described his attitude toward saving for later in life:

> I felt like everything was temporary. Like I've—and to this day this is true. I've never contributed to me, um, to my pension fund. Till to this day. It feels—even though I'm 40. I never did it—um. I just—I never did it and I—I've always felt like, "Why should I be doing that? I'm never gonna get to the point of using it."

Such tales are common in the lives of men of my generation, as many men lived without abandon, spending their savings, foregoing their promising and successful careers, and not planning for the future, only to discover after 1996 that they would survive this death sentence. Why were they to think or act any differently when all they witnessed was death?

The Grim Reaper: Death Is All Around

For Hal, who is now married to his childhood sweetheart, the experiences of death in his social circle are indicative of many of the men of the AIDS Generation:

> I was in San Francisco hoping no one would die there. And then they all died. Then I moved to Provincetown and they all died.

Later in our discussion, Hal described how this part of his life was characterized by ongoing death while he himself was struggling to stay alive:

> There was a real intense surge of death in like '88, '89 and my friend Patrick, when he died I was holding his feet. I sort of chose—I had so much

fear about death and the dying process that I started choosing to be present at people's death and had the great fortune of being honored to be there by the families because I wanted to demystify that because the deaths of my childhood, my mother was lost at sea, my grandmother killed herself in a garage, I didn't see dead bodies and there was just something—you know in our society we put death in a hospital and we don't look at it. So I was present for these deaths and it was a profound experience for me to watch people pass because they were mostly gentle passings ultimately at the end. There was an exhalation and it was peaceful. And the way they looked right after they'd died. The stress was gone from their faces. They looked peaceful. They looked—so it removed a lot of fear. It didn't make the loss any easier. I mean the loss was still horrible and painful but I think it helped me with my survival.

Hal further described the extent of his losses to AIDS and how these conditions extended to his work environment at GMHC:

Acquaintances, over 100 because I worked at GMHC. One guy—I had a couple of guys die right in the office, one died at the copier. He was copying and he just keeled over, so a lot. Close friends maybe 10, one assisted suicide.

The experiences that Hal describes are the conditions that we, all gay men of the AIDS Generation, were facing at that time. In a recent episode of *American Masters,* David Geffen, the music, film, and theater producer and founder of DreamWorks, was portrayed. One powerful clip shows Geffen receiving the AIDS Project Los Angeles Commitment to Life Award in 1992. During this speech Geffen emotionally recalls refusing to remove the card of his friend, choreographer Michael Bennett, from his Rolodex, and how this one card had quickly become 341 cards all held together by a rubber band. For me personally, the loss was limited to the five significant men I named in the first chapter. In the course of writing this book, I had a large nautical star tattooed on the center of my right arm. Around the center star and in tribute are five smaller red stars representing the five men in my life who I have lost to AIDS.

For Ralph, who had moved from Salt Lake City to San Francisco, where he worked as a bartender on Castro Street, the experience of death was front and center:

Every week *The Bay,* or there were two papers, *The Sentinel* and *The Bay Area Reporter*, and they—I don't believe *The Sentinel* as much, but *The Bay*

Area Reporter always had the funeral page, you know, two or three pages of people that died that week. It was terrible.

When I asked him if he knew many of those in the local areas newspaper, Ralph indicated:

Yeah, well, I mean, because I was the bartender, you know. I always thought of the bartender as being the gay cheerleader. Um, I knew a lot of them, yeah, it was pretty horrible. That, again, was the holocaust thing, you know, watching everybody die in front of you knowing that, whoa, God, I hope they get a good picture of me when I'm on there.

Ralph and his partner at the time, who has since died, moved from Salt Lake City to San Francisco after their diagnoses. Throughout the course of our discussion, Ralph returned many times over to the image of the Holocaust, drawing parallels between the AIDS epidemic in the gay community in San Francisco and the experience of the 12 million who died in World War II.

I mean, San Francisco was wonderful. I never thought of it as ghetto, but somehow I always related to the Holocaust and that idea of gathering and then into the ghetto, and then eventually, you know, it was into the camps, I guess. . . .

The voice of Antoine provides yet anther take on a very similar situation, yet under different circumstances and within a different social context. Recall that Antoine had developed his circle of friends—his family—in his adolescence as a gay man in Prospect Park, Brooklyn. In 1982, 3 years before his own diagnosis, and at age 23, Antoine began to experience the loss that would characterize his life for close to two decades as he recalled the first AIDS-related death, as well as the associated confusion and discrimination at that time:

A friend of ours who danced for Alvin Ailey was sitting in Lucien's place. And we were all planning that night, that next night, to go to Paradise Garage. And he said, "Look, listen, guys. I don't feel well. And I'm gonna go home." And the next day, that Saturday at 2:00, he called us up and said, "I can't go. Something is wrong with me and I don't know what it is. And I need you guys to come and look at me." And we was like, "Look at you? Why?" And he was Perry Ellis, the designer's, assistant. And when we got to his house, we were just in awe because he had all the purple spots. On his face. And we didn't know. You know, my first intention was, "You either got a bad case of the chicken pox or the mumps." You know, but—but in the meantime, you still gotta go to—you go to the hospital. And when we took him to Methodist Hospital, they basically thought he had cancer. And that was my first introduction to makeup because a friend of his that was in the fashion world said to cover up those spots, use this Derma Blend. And then we realized, he says, "But guys, it's not just on the face." And he pulled up his pants. So my first introduction was—because he still wanted to go out, he would say, "Well, you know, I'll lay on the bed, and you apply this Derma Blend to my entire body before we leave." And that was it. But we all thought it was cancer. Well, it was so ironic because he lasted 21 days....And that was my—that was a horrific experience. Because it took five—we had to go to five undertakers before the fifth one would take his body. And he made it plain to us there's no need to buy any clothes. We're just going to wrap him up in a sheet and burn him.

In *AIDS Doctors: Voices From the Epidemic* (2000), Ronald Bayer and Gerald Oppenheimer provide an oral history of the experiences of doctors working with AIDS patients during the onset of the epidemic. The experiences of the doctors they interviewed who were in the frontline battle with the disease complement and further illustrate the experiences of the men of the AIDS Generation. Like the men with whom I spoke, these doctors witnessed abundant and devastating amounts of death. At institutions like San Francisco General Hospital and St. Vincent's Hospital in the Greenwich Village section of New York City, it was conceivable to experience 20 or more AIDS deaths in a period of a month. Reflecting on this reality for the oral history project described in the book, one physician described her role as "a travel agent for death" (p. 271).

St. Vincent's Hospital is where my partner Robert died in my arms on April 9, 1994. The hospital closed its doors due to bankruptcy in 2010; it has been speculated that this site, which was not only a focal point on 9/11 but also ground zero for the AIDS epidemic, had this financial meltdown because HIV treatment advances had put them out of the "AIDS business." The editors of *OUT* magazine (Armstrong, 2010) paid tribute to the site by interviewing those who were present on the AIDS ward of the hospital in those years prior to the implementation of ART. Mark Chambers, a veteran of the AIDS ward, described it as follows:

The early years are still like a horror movie that you have nightmares over, and then you realize it wasn't real, except it was. At St. Vincent's you didn't get inside the hospital—you got into the emergency room, and that's where your friends were lined up on gurneys. My most vivid memory is of my best friend—who I had gotten a call about 12 hours earlier—still lying there, wasting and close to death, along with many other AIDS patients, waiting for attention. It was a scene of total helplessness on the part of both the patients and the staff. (p. 92)

There is no reason to recount the enormous losses faced by gay men in the first two decades of AIDS. This has been abundantly documented in the epidemiological, behavioral, and medical literature and has been recounted in numerous documentaries. My point of reference to the realities at San Francisco General and St. Vincent's is merely to provide a backdrop and context for the world in which the men of the AIDS Generation were living and to provide a framing for the meaning that their diagnosis held at this particular historical moment. Put simply, death was all around, and they too had become victims of the virus that could soon terminate their lives.

In recalling their lives as HIV-positive individuals, the men with whom I spoke clearly articulated the loss they witnessed and experienced during the early days of AIDS, while simultaneously managing their conditions, which without any significant breakthrough in treatment would lead to their own demise. Many had to care for those who were dying while they themselves were also dying. This is no more evident than in the story told by Antoine, who described in detail the loss of the family of friends he had developed in Prospect Park. Describing the death of one of his friends, Antoine again fell back on the image of the cocoon to describe how he managed the loss and death he was experiencing and how he and his inner circle cared for each other:

Like I said to a person 3 years ago, I basically went into a cocoon because if I would have actually thought consciously what I was doing, I don't think I would have been able to handle it because so many of my friends were dying and I was attending funerals left and right and this and that. So now, like I say to people, death has very little effect on me because I've seen so much of it. I mean one of the horrific experiences I had to experience was when my friend Albert was in Lenox Hill Hospital, and me and my cousin Lucien had to—and my chief petty officer—because he was also gay— made arrangements for me because we were in his room, and I witnessed the nurse putting his plate on the floor by the door because she didn't want to come into his room. And I'm like, "Well, how is he supposed to get that plate when he's too weak to get out of bed?" So me and my cousin Lucien had devised a schedule that at 11:30 he would meet me at Battery Park. We would drive up to Lenox Hill Hospital, make sure he had his lunch, come back and feed him for dinner. Because his parents lived in Alabama. And he had no one here.

Antoine's story is replete with loss to AIDS. He recalls 40 members of his inner social circle, his gay family, including himself, who were HIV positive when he first became aware of his HIV status in 1985. On New Year's Eve in 1991, at a loft party in Greenwich Village, only 20 of those 40 were still alive. In 2012, that number was reduced to three. And for Jackson, experiencing the loss was situated within his circle of five. The five scoured over the early reports of the epidemic in the local area papers and any other documents they could ascertain, searching for clues and answers. At the conclusion of that story, Jackson states, "And of the five people there, I'm one of the two that are still alive."

Long Island–born John, who speaks openly about his status to high school groups, also recalled the loss he experienced in his social circle while sharing the story of his own seroconversion. Recalling hearing the news that he too was living with HIV and being assured that he too would die, John said:

And I walked out of there with tears in my eyes. And Peter [parner at the time] looked at me, and said, "Oh, no." I said, "I got it." And he said, "What do you want to do?" I said, "I've gotta get some vodka, and some coke, some pot. I just can't deal with this." By then I had been to hundreds of funerals, you know, oh. Many, many, many funerals, and had been to hospitals and watched these people die these horrible deaths. Guys, you know, younger than me who were in great shape. And, uh, you know, so I knew I'd be—I would make the 30 because it was only 2 weeks away, but I said—figured that would be the end of it.

For some others, the loss extended beyond their friendship circles to their partners and lovers, as was the case for Gianni, who recalled in painstaking detail the loss of his partner and how he had to manage the death process of his partner while maintaining his own viability:

It's horrible, it's horrible, it's horrible. I had no support. I have a few people at work who knew who are my friends. I had my mother who was very helpful at that time, um, in that Italian mother sort of way. Um, I had David's [his partner's] cousin, I had our friend, Ellen, who we were very close with, was very helpful. Um, but mostly—and then his family, which was not—were not very helpful because, you know—they were not very helpful, but I managed this on my own. And, um, 'cause I had to. And then he died. And then he—then—then one day I was getting dressed for work and I was waiting for the home health care aide to come sit with him, and he couldn't breathe.... So, um, ambulance came, went to the hospital, spent the night sleeping with him in the bed, he was being morphined up, Ellen was sleeping on the floor, woke up the next morning, he was—his mother and father and sister were coming from Jersey, and then he just got up from the bed as I was holding him and gasped and then died. That was horrible. That was horrible. And that's it. I just have this blur for the next like decade after that.

The loss experienced by the men of the AIDS Generation crossed all aspects of their lives—friends, lovers, acquaintances, work colleagues, family members. No one was immune from the devastation. These losses live vividly in the memories of the men with whom I spoke. Perhaps more than any other, it is John's recollection of his losses that best captures the extent of this devastation experienced by the men of the AIDS Generation. During this portion of our conversation, John cried without any hesitation as he recalled the numerous losses of his life, inspired by first recalling the death of his ensuing partner, his husband, Rafael:

Rafael—he moved in with me, and, uh, we were married. We had a commitment ceremony in 1995. My parents threw it at their house, and we had 250 people, and, uh, and he died in 2002, and I was with him when he died, and that was very painful because he was only 40. [Crying]

And I had when I was growing up, a guy who was like—I considered my, um, like Walter, he died of AIDS. I wasn't with him. And then Colin was this older guy who got me my first job, who got me my first suit, um, he died of AIDS. Um, you know, my boss who I was very, very close with, Norman, who was like my gay mother, Walter was like my gay father, this guy was like my gay brother, and Frank was my best friend; they all died. All those people that were supposed to be with me for the rest of my life.

The four voices reflected previously, those of Hal, Antoine, Gianni, and John, provide insight into the contexts and circumstances in which the men of the AIDS Generation were living and trying to remain healthy and viable. All 15 men recalled experiences of loss and death. None escaped the effects of the Grim Reaper, and the abundance of such stories of loss could fill this entire volume. And each lived with the constant and looming cloud over their heads and their friends' heads, as Patrick, who eventually moved to New York City, recalls:

> And calling each other on the phone: "I got this thing on my—I got a bruise, it doesn't look like KS, it could be, I don't know what it is...." "Are you going to go to the doctor?" "I don't know." We did that a lot. Almost every other night.

I have recently shown that aging HIV-positive men, those who are members of the AIDS Generation, experience posttraumatic stress disorder (PTSD) at higher rates than even those who witnessed the event of 9/11 or any other disaster (Halkitis, Kupprat, et al., 2013). In short, the AIDS epidemic has been our natural disaster, which has left an indelible scar in our lives. But singly and as a population we have shown resilience and continue to forge ahead. Our collective and individual trauma due to the AIDS epidemic as well as our will to continue with our lives was expressed with pinpoint precision by Jackson, who was raised Baptist in Washington, DC, in explaining his reaction at his father's funeral, which functioned as a trigger igniting his emotions:

> So but when my father died, I think I had convinced myself that I had packed away a lot of—of my feelings and—and sadness and the trauma. And I wasn't going to the theater often because I would just not go. I just— my mind would wander. I wouldn't watch the show. I would think about, you know, just the whole experience of being in the lobby and sitting down in the theater seats just brought me back there. I just avoided it. And going through the experience with my father, his dying—because his bodily systems shutting down one by one and started to lose his mind, and it was a slow process.
>
> Getting pneumonia, hearing the words "Bactrim" and "Septra" and hearing the death rattle. And this happened in slow motion compared to what my experience had been. So it was—you know, it wasn't like—but I—I remember, and I was supporting my mom going through all that, too. But I would go out to the parking lot because I was by myself sitting in the car, it would just erupt. Not for my father but all the memories. They only just scratched the surface, and they would come flooding back.
>
> And they were all so vivid and so terrible that I realized my life is going to be a struggle between, you know, honoring the fallen soldiers and the memory of the time and ACT UP and what I'm holding in my heart and trying to find some measure of peace within myself so that I can walk

away—you know, live my life. You know, and that—but that's just going to be life.

The experiences of death due to AIDS seem like an endless pit for all of us as, noted in John's recollections:

It [Mark's death] started this process, Frank died, the hairdresser died when I—after I got sober; I was with him. Yeah, uh, yup, um-hmm. Frank died. My boss [Norman] died. Um, my—my—my partner died. [Crying] He—he died in 2002.

Such conditions would characterize all of our lives, all of the gay men who came of age right before or during the first decade of AIDS. To this day, the three Aprils of 1992, 1993, and 1994 are the darkest periods of my life. I lost my father on April 20, 1992. Then, AIDS stole from me my best friend Tony (April 1, 1993) and my partner Robert (April 9, 1994).

Conclusions

Finding out that one is living with HIV is a life-altering event for anyone. This is perhaps even more profound for the men of the AIDS Generation, or for any person diagnosed in the first two decades of the disease, a time of limited hope. This pivotal life moment continues to be clearly present in the consciousness of the men of the AIDS Generation, shown in the words of Ralph: "Well, there are some experiences that you remember in your life, you know, falling in love for the first time, or you know, different things. I always remember that."

All of the men with whom I spoke, despite the fact that they had experienced life-altering events, continued on their life paths, either through the enactment of active, health-seeking or avoidant, destructive strategies, which was all they could do in that period of their lives that followed their diagnoses. After the pause passed, many of the men proceeded with their lives, attempting to normalize existence and determine how to stay healthy and stay alive. Normalizing, focusing on living, taking care of oneself, being in relation to others, and triumphing are the essentials to surviving AIDS, according to Julie Barroso (1997).

In Jonathan Demme's harrowing 1993 film *Philadelphia,* we are introduced to Andrew Beckett, who is living with HIV. Early in the film, Beckett travels from his high-powered law firm to his doctor's office to receive his blood test results. After sitting in the waiting room surrounded by those who are suffering from a multitude of opportunist infections, Beckett returns to the demands of his career. He, like so many, had no choice but to continue on his path. I walked my partner Robert, whose body had been ravaged by progressive multifocal leukoencephalopathy (PML), which paralyzed one side of his body, to see this film during the last few months of his life, providing him some sense of normality, a factor deemed critical in the lives of those living with HIV (Barroso, 1997; Crossley, 1999).

After this initial period of shock and awe regarding the news of their HIV status or the advanced status of their HIV disease, many of the men of the AIDS Generation described moving forward with their lives, trying to manage their disease and live with a sense of dignity. Such reactions are not uncommon among those who have received a terminal diagnosis. Michele Davies (1997) suggests that for some individuals receiving a diagnosis of a terminal disease, as was the case with AIDS prior to 1996, there exists a sense that living (or not dying) is a possibility. In the years that followed their diagnoses, the men of the AIDS Generation moved on with their lives, calling on a multitude of coping strategies to ensure their survival. Some of these approaches were active and health seeking, whereas others were avoidant and health compromising. However, what they did to survive and how they managed to survive provides us all with great insight into the resilience of the human spirit.

The significance of being diagnosed with HIV or AIDS cannot be underestimated, especially in the first two decades of the epidemic in the United States and in the population of gay men. For the men of the AIDS Generation, this life-altering event so early in their adulthood shaped the path of their lives for the next 20 or more years and continues to shape their lives to this day. The AIDS epidemic defined a generation of gay men, my generation, and became a significant historical moment in the life of New York City. In 2012, Sam Roberts, urban correspondent for *The New York Times*, defined the 50 most significant and important objects in the history of New York. One of these is the AIDS button, with the image of "SILENCE=DEATH," developed by the artistic collective Gran Fury and, which became the centerpiece of the ACT UP movement (Gran Fury & Cohen, 2011). Of this historical object, Roberts (2012, p. 6 online) writes:

In 1982, 752 cases of a mysterious and fatal illness that would be called Acquired Immune Deficiency Syndrome were reported in New York City. By 2010, nearly 170,000 cases had been diagnosed. Over 30 years, the illness devastated whole communities even as it served as a focal point for the gay rights movement, especially Act Up, which campaigned vigorously against the government's slow response to the epidemic. The city's health department describes New York as the nation's epicenter of H.I.V./AIDS. Today, about 100,000 New Yorkers are living with the disease, thanks to advanced medicines. But it is still the third leading cause of death for New Yorkers between the ages of 35 and 54.

I have two ACT UP buttons, one that was mine and one that was Robert's, that I keep prominently displayed in a shadow box in my apartment. As a population of gay men and despite more than 30 years of trauma, we have moved on. But there is never a day that I want to forget where we were 30 years ago, nor that for the last 30 years, "most of us in the age of AIDS have thought of the enemy as HIV itself" (Rotello, 1997, p. 4).

CHAPTER 4 | Surviving AIDS

Strategies for Managing a Life With HIV

ALL OF THE MEN of the AIDS Generation lived through the ravages of AIDS and survived to tell me their stories in 2012. Their experiences for the last 20 or more years illustrate a complicated and demanding life journey beautifully articulated by Antoine, who, you will recall, described himself as "a 52-year-old African American man, who is actually gay, born this way":

> I've been at the worst of this virus, and now I'm in the golden years of this virus. This virus has taken me halfway around the world, and I'm still here.

As was shown previously, the men of the AIDS Generation experienced the news of their own HIV diagnoses, and expected mortality, while simultaneously witnessing decimation in their own social circles and in the gay community at large. This life condition was true for all of the men, whether it was front and center, as it was for Jackson, who was a dancer in New York City and who defined the theater community as "ground zero of the AIDS epidemic in New York," or more removed as it was for Patrick, as he shuttled between Nevada and Texas during this time. For the men of the AIDS Generation, this ongoing onslaught of the AIDS epidemic defined their formative years of emerging and young adulthood. In fact, this emotional cacophony was true even for those like Eddie, who had developed a mythological understanding that gay-related immune deficiency (GRID) was a condition confined to white gay men and, as a result, he was somehow immune from this disease.

AIDS altered the lives of the men of my generation. All of us, whether we now are HIV-positive or HIV-negative middle-aged men, were halted in our tracks when AIDS became an ever-present reality in our lives. We were derailed from the process of emerging into adulthood with hopes and dreams, prevented from resolving the emotional conflicts of young adulthood, and forced to face ongoing illness and death straight on, a situation that was quite unnatural for men of our age.

For all humans, the journey of life is complex and fraught with challenges. For the men of the AIDS Generation, the disease exacerbated these life challenges, undermining "normal" development. In this chapter, we examine and frame this disruption of normal life processes and consider the biological, psychological, and social strategies and processes that the men of the AIDS Generation enacted to survive. Such approaches were informed by the men's attention to their whole selves and likely driven by a will to live and triumph over HIV—their spirit. I also present strategies in the forms of use of alcohol and other drugs as well as reliance on sex as means of framing these approaches in a somewhat less judgmental manner.

The Unexpected Life Crisis

In his seminal work, *Identity and the Life Cycle* (1980, p. 53), psychologist Erik H. Erikson states the following with regard to health and growth:

> Whenever we try to understand growth, it is well to remember the epigenetic principle, which is derived from the growth of the organism in utero. Somewhat generalized, this principle states that anything that grows has a ground plan, and out of the ground plan the first parts arise, each part having its time and special ascendancy, until all the parts have arisen to form a functioning whole.

This epigenetic approach (Erikson, 1980; Erikson & Erikson, 1997) postulates a series of life stages that inform the development of our psychological and social well-being. Erikson posits that throughout our lifetimes and across the spectrum of ages, we struggle through a series of conflicts— emotional conflicts that characterize the milestones along the developmental continuum—and that the resolutions of these conflicts or tensions inform our psychosocial development. These developmental stages span from cradle to grave, and the effective handling of the emotional conflicts within each stage of development allows us to move forward in the formation of our integrated whole. In the absence of a healthy resolution, we are saddled with the emotional burdens of that developmental stage throughout the course of our lives, and they become a burden we carry as we emerge into the ensuing developmental periods. In addition to syntonic and dystonic forces that characterize associated developmental periods, each of these identity conflicts is characterized by an overriding existential question and a significant relationship. For the infant ages 0 to 2, it is "Can I trust the world?" and the significant relationship is that with the mother. For those in later adulthood ages, 65 and older, the individual grapples with the question "Is it acceptable to have been me?" and the significant relationship is that with the world around him.

For the men of the AIDS Generation, the HIV epidemic interfered with the struggle of many men to resolve emotional conflicts and to form an integrated whole. For all of these men, the epidemic came at a time when they were emerging into adulthood and beginning to make their places in the world after leaving their homes and families and setting out to advance their education, to launch their careers, and/or to find someone to love. In the framing of Eriksonian identity theory, these men at the time of their diagnosis, like all young adults, were grappling with existential questions of "Can I love?" and "Can I make my life count?" However, while the men of the AIDS Generation were grappling with these emotional struggles, as all young adults were, they also were suddenly, unexpectedly, and without any warning confronted with AIDS. Their significant relationships with partners and lovers, like those of Hal and Antoine, were undone because of the death that was permeating their social circles, because their lovers were dying in their arms, and because love became synonymous with death for so many men. At the same time, others, like Kerry who had charted a course of a career and forged relationships with colleagues and workmates, abandoned these opportunities either because they were too ill to work or because they feared that time was limited and wanted to make the most of what was left. Recall the "myth of two." Christopher, who traces his seroconversion to a casual encounter in Jersey City, summarized this thinking about his life after his HIV diagnosis as follows:

> That I had like 5 or 6 years to live. That I would have to change my whole career. That I would never have sex again. That I was gonna die like this slow and painful death. Um, there were a whole host of—I mean, damaged goods, you know, you're not datable if you're outside—you know, not in a relationship. Um, yeah, it was—it was really, really, really rough.

To the reader, my peripatetic journey into Eriksonian theory may seem out of context or seem like an unnecessary diversion from the basic premise of this work. However, these concepts are critical for two main reasons. First, when examining the strategies for survival that the men of the AIDS Generation enacted, it is important to remember and to be reminded that these men were confronting not only HIV and all its complications but also the "normal" developmental challenges facing most individuals as they transitioned from adolescence into young and full adulthood. These transitions are difficult for many and some fail in charting effective life courses, but for the men of the AIDS Generation these challenges were saddled and obstructed by the conditions AIDS had created in their lives, which interfered with normal developmental processes. It is in this regard that one must consider the strategies for surviving HIV that the men employed—strategies for survival that superseded the demands of normal human development and the resolution of the identity crises that characterize this period of life. Second, as we come to know the men as middle aged in the ensuing chapters, an Eriksonian framing provides a lens for understanding the emotional lives of these now-older men, conditions first set in place by the inability to fully and completely resolve the emotional conflicts of a younger age due to the onslaught of AIDS, and moreover how the healthy resolution of the syntonic and dystonic forces of middle age are associated with a reexamination of the past (Erikson, Erikson, & Kivinick, 1986). The men of the AIDS Generation did not experience the luxury of life as young adults, a condition that informs their lives to this day, a condition that is quite evident as these men, having survived death at a younger age, seek to understand their lives and legacies as middle-aged men.

Attending to the Whole

Throughout the course of my career I have framed my understanding of HIV and other health conditions using the holism of a biopsychosocial framework (Halkitis, 2009, 2010a; Halkitis Wolitski, et al., 2013). In this view, HIV is more than an infection with a pathogen. Rather, HIV, like all other illnesses, transgresses the physical, emotional, and social well-being of the person. Approaching HIV disease using a biopsychosocial lens allows us to understand and recognize that HIV-infected individuals, like the men of the AIDS Generation, are more than disease vessels, but multidimensional complex individuals. Living with HIV has enormous implications in all aspects of the person's life, not solely on his immune system. In effect, disentangling why some succeed in managing their disease while others fail requires that we attend to the multifaceted nature of HIV-positive individuals and the strategies they enact to address their biological/physical, psychological, and social well-being.

HIV is an illness that dilutes the physical, emotional, and social well-being of the man living with the disease. Although management of the infection is absolutely crucial, treatment of that pathogen alone is insufficient in addressing the total health of the HIV-infected man and ensuring his survival, as noted in the words of this 57-year-old Project Gold study participant: "Well, I have a really strong belief that HIV, it's more about health, general health, and overall health than anything specifically related to HIV." For another Project Gold participant, a 55-year-old Black man, HIV was the impetus for him to begin to attend to the well-being of his whole self:

> HIV took me to a whole—a whole new level. It took me to a whole new level and, uh, I don't, in a way, and um, I had to think of a positive way. HIV saved my life.... I'm doing support groups now, um, and trying to find a better way to live. But, um, it—it led to me into a world that I—I never thought I would be in.

This notion of caring for the whole is one that was evident in the voices of the men of the AIDS Generation. Each spoke of specific strategies that implicated the physical, emotional, and social domains, but they also spoke articulately about attending to the entirety of their being—to the connection between mind, body, and spirit. This attendance to the whole was evident in my interaction with Christopher, which I report in its entirety to demonstrate the logic pattern utilized by Christopher in attending to all aspects of his well-being:

> CHRISTOPHER: It was that—that, I always call it that—I guess it was sort of a panic state and you spend the majority of your time trying to find out and do as many things as you can about it.
> PERRY: About your disease?
> CHRISTOPHER: About your disease.
> PERRY: And what is—when—and when you say try to do as many things, what do you mean?
> CHRISTOPHER: Find a support group, talk to other people, get information. And that was before the Internet.
> PERRY: Yep.

CHRISTOPHER: Um, find a doctor, find—like, it was like I have to get this done and I have to get this done now.

PERRY: So it sounds to me like you were trying to control it by doing all of these things.

CHRISTOPHER: A little bit, yeah. I think it was just this panic, you know, like, "Oh, my God, oh, my God, I need to know. I need to know. I need to do this. I need to do this. I need to do this. I need to do this because I have to stay"—you know.

PERRY: So where did you go for the support group?

CHRISTOPHER: There was a support group in Maplewood, New Jersey, at the time, and while it was helpful overall, it was for affected, infected, men, women—IVD users.

PERRY: Right.

CHRISTOPHER: And I think a—a good half of those people were IV drug users so I didn't get everything out of it that I could have, but I did meet one of like my best friends ever, who passed away a bunch of years ago, which was worth the whole experience to me. And he was the only one I talked to subsequent to moving away from here.

PERRY: Where did you find the doctor?

CHRISTOPHER: Um, actually, my partner used to go—his GP was the first doctor I went to. And he said that—he said—he goes, "I will gladly see you whenever you need to, but I think"—he's like, "I think you should go to a specialist."

PERRY: Yeah.

CHRISTOPHER: Um, I—but he took my first T-cell count and reran the test just to make sure that everything—

PERRY: Right.

CHRISTOPHER: —was correct. And, um, but he suggested like—and then, um, Bruce [partner] had friends that were involved with the Long Island Association for AIDS Care at the time. So I was hooked up as a client there and, um, I wound up getting a caseworker and I wound up going to a clinic in Freeport for a number of years, until I switched doctors and now I go to a guy at North Shore Hospital.

PERRY: Okay.

CHRISTOPHER: Um, but, yeah, like—like I—like I said I was getting my and, um, you know, just getting my regular visits, get all my blood work, that sort of stuff. I have a caseworker, um, and because the caseworker I had liked me so much, he even got me like a buddy that I talk to often, um, still.

PERRY: To this day.

CHRISTOPHER: Yeah. I mean, it's—not as much because he moved to Georgia a number of years. He was quite a bit older than me. He probably could be my dad, but—

PERRY: Okay.

CHRISTOPHER: He, um, he was nice. Just very—very nice, very generous.

PERRY: Okay.

CHRISTOPHER: And, um, um, had a good, you know, support. And then wound up—somebody suggested that, um, because I had moved to Long Island to move in with Daniel since 1992, and I had gone to an intake at Body Positive, and I think it was 6 months before I was in a group.

PERRY: Body Positive on Fulton Street?

Christopher: Yeah.

PERRY: Yeah.

CHRISTOPHER: Um, and then I was put in and enrolled to a group.

What we see in this interaction with Christopher is that attendance to both his physical and socio-emotional well-being was how he first conceptualized his management of AIDS. However, his strategies were also based on guesses and suppositions of what would truly prove to be the most effective approach. Indeed, for the men of the AIDS Generation, approaches to handling their condition in the period prior to the implementation of effective treatments required truly innovative thinking and occasional guesswork. It required attending to the messages being sent by their bodies, management of emotional states in a time laden with confusion and chaos, and support from systems wide and varied to cope with this life-threatening disease. And it is along these three domains—the physical, emotional, and social self—that the men of the AIDS Generation described their strategies for survival, with the underlying belief that attention to the whole would yield the most powerful results. To follow, I delineate the strategies enacted by the men of the AIDS Generation that attended to the physical, emotional, and social domains of their lives, and which likely led to their survival.

The Physical Self

Attendance to one's body characterized the first set of strategies enacted by the men of the AIDS Generation. This took the form of enacting of health programs, experimentation with a variety of therapeutics, and elimination of behaviors that were deemed to compromise physical health.

Caring for one's physical self permeated the story that Patrick shared. A professional dancer and choreographer, Patrick has attended to the needs of his physical body throughout the course of his infection and in a variety of manners. This approach to surviving HIV is very evident in his lifestyle to this day:

> I get up every morning. I teach from 6:00 in the morning until 3:00 in the afternoon. I am a fitness professional. I do health and fitness, I personal train, I run a gym. And I come home. I eat dinner quickly because I need to get food in my stomach and then I'm in bed by 9:30.

This pattern of physical self-care was evident in a variety of forms in Patrick's life, including his eating habits, inspired by his boyfriend at the time, shortly after his HIV diagnosis:

> And then I was with my new boyfriend, when I decided to live in Houston, in Galveston area, fell in love with an older, Jewish guy [Melvin]. Seven years older again, and negative. And we decided to live together. Very health conscious, very—juice every morning, took all kinds of this—and I think he saw me as I'm going to take this 27-year-old guy who has this problem and I'm going to make him get away from these cheeseburgers and stop drinking all the milk and drink carrot juice and do this and this and this and also he has a morbid fear of doctors too.

Care of the physical self for Patrick also translated into a close relationship and careful negotiation with his doctors throughout the course of his disease:

> And I kind of knew that I liked my doctors, I needed my doctors. And I would kind of get mad at him sometimes. He [Melvin] would say, "Those doctors are going to kill you." And I would say, "No, they're not because I'm smart enough to—I know I have to bring to the table—I'm not going to let them dictate to me what they're going to do. If I don't like something, I'm going to tell them because I know my body. They don't know—they know the technical stuff about my body, but I know what it feels like."

Caring for the physical self through partnership with his doctor was and is also true for New York area–born and –raised Gianni ("I bring up studies with my doctor even now") and for John (who, you will recall, built up his body as an adolescent to avoid being bullied, a physique he carries to this day), who forged a close working relationship with his health care provider and who stayed informed of the HIV health literature:

> Early on one of the doctors I had had said to me—because I studied it and looked into things and got involved in trials and the GP 160 and was telling her all these things I was doing and finding out. And she said one of the wisest things I had ever heard, which was, "This is your disease. It's a new disease; we hardly know anything about it. You gotta be more informed than I am."
>
> And it was very smart. And I realized that even to this day that I got to know about this disease because a lot of these doctors that—I go to a clinic and they don't know sometimes. I'm more up on it and contemporary on the disease than they are. And I gotta be. I gotta stay abreast of it.

It was clear from my interactions with Patrick that attention to his body was how he managed his disease. However, he also perceived the social and emotional benefits of his actions, although the voice of the physical self is the one that resonates the loudest. With his peers as part of the focus group, Patrick described his self-care as follows:

> From the very beginning, I didn't go into denial, I accepted it pretty well, but my thing was I got to keep what makes my body happy going. And I was dancing professionally then and choreographing and working all the time. And I had to keep that up no matter what because I found that I can't sit still. I move all the—that's just what makes me happy.

Grasping for Any Treatment Option

Prior to 1996, no amount of juice or healthy eating or even the early HIV antivirals such as AZT and 3TC seemed to be powerful enough to deter the infection and keep it at bay. So, many, like my partner Robert, attempted to care for the physical self through the use of complementary therapies, in his case, egg yolks and soybeans (AL721). Others "medicated" with Kombucha mushrooms, and others with bitter melon and assorted other nontraditional, non-Western approaches. Robert looked with great pride on the May 30, 1989, *Village Voice* cover story of yet another such treatment, Compound Q (Kua-lou, or GLQ244) (Goldstein & Massa, 1989), which was made from the root of a Chinese cucumber, and which, like all others, proved not to be the miracle for which we were hoping. These efforts on Robert's part were also a means for managing his own health—knowing as much as he could, as described earlier by Gianni and John.

Other approaches, including meditation, acupuncture, Reiki, and treatments with crystals, were provided by agencies like GMHC to help improve the health and well-being of the walking dead. Some ate only macrobiotic food. Everyone who was affected or infected was grasping for every possibility to beat the virus. The desperation in our hearts was debilitating and deafening. Hal summed it up as follows: "So I mean I was, if I could have shoved a crystal up my ass that would have healed me, I would have done it. I mean that's how it was." In a similar mode, Patrick described one other approach to care that he underwent with his friends early in his own diagnosis and in the early days of the epidemic:

> My friend at that time had gotten a job up in Vegas. He invited me to come up to Vegas because he heard there was this secret thing, a cure nobody knew about. It was eight guys. We stayed in one house. It was patented; it was going to be. They were these little boxes and the boxes emitted a kind of frequency. It was too high; you couldn't hear it. Because the person that had invented these, he had done research and he figured out that the HIV virus was in a crystalline form. So this high-frequency sound, if we were around them, would shatter the crystalline form and it would be attacked that way. So we said, "Hey, why not."

It does not appear that any of these treatments hurt us, but they did not truly help. That breakthrough would come in 1996. Hal reflected on recently rereading Michael Callen's book, *Surviving AIDS*, and how that reminded him of everything he and others undertook in the early days of AIDS to deter the infection and build physical strength:

> Yeah. I met him once, but I'm rereading it and I'm just like, "Wow." It just takes you back to that point and you know—well like, and people were trying—the PWA Coalition—I had first gone there—people were trying mushrooms and I went to Arizona to Sedona and saw shamans and faith healers and I mean in my desperation I think we were drinking our own urine at one point. I mean—oxygen therapy.

For Antoine, the treatment of choice was interferon, which was utilized to treat HIV in the early days of the epidemic. Despite some helpful effects (Rivero, Fraga, Cancio, Cuervo, & Lopez-Saura, 1997), interferon also has been shown to perhaps have exacerbated the epidemic and created some harm (Yabrov, 2000). Again, this was a treatment administered at a time of little hope, so the good may have outweighed the bad when there were no other options. For Antoine, the struggle was not only to remain alive but also to access this treatment for himself and for his social circle. To this end, Antoine was savvy and made use of his membership in the U.S. Coast Guard to transport the treatment, which he then was able to also administer to himself, despite the fact that he had limited economic means to purchase the drug:

> Whoo. Whoo. I mean I could never forget using my Coast Guard military uniform—to travel from New York to Mayport, Florida, to get interferon because they would not search my bag if I was in full military uniform. For me and my friends because my friend, um, Daniel, who lives in London, had a lover who was also a twin that was both gay. And they opened a clothing store in the South Street Seaport. And Daniel's lover—I believe his name was George—the family were quite well off, and the father, like you reading that *Times* paper, for some, some way or another, he found this doctor in Mayport, Florida, that would dispense—interferon. So I would get on a plane and get a 120-day supply of these little pills—that they had, for like—and his father [coughs], excuse me—he paid for all of us. Me, Daniel, Lucien, Abert, Brenda, um, Christian, Jadden—I mean all 20 of us. And I was looking at this man, and he was like, "You know, these are my two sons, and I love them no matter what." To Florida, 6 hours there and 6 hours back, don't worry about it.

Ultimately, all of the men of the AIDS Generation simply needed to wait until 1996, when the course of the epidemic radically changed in the face of effective combinations of therapies. Prior to that point, many were grasping for any treatment possibility or, as noted in the words of Jackson, simply trying to remain physically healthy until those treatments would arrive: "I just thought I'm gonna do everything I can to buy myself another 2 years and maybe there'll be another medication and maybe there'll be something else coming over the next horizon."

Healthy Sex

For some of the men of the AIDS Generation, taking care of the physical self also required realignment with their sexual behavior. Early in the epidemic, there was much heated debate and controversy regarding safer sex practices and the transmission of HIV, which Larry Kramer perfectly depicts in his play *The Normal Heart* (2000).

Even after it was established that one act alone could confer infection, and the notions that the amount, number, or frequency of sexual partners were not quite correct in establishing a causal path between sexual behavior and seroconversion, other contradictions regarding sex and infectivity emerged. This was most pronounced with regard to the matter of reinfection—whether one could be infected more than once with HIV, which would lead to infection with mosaic and more virulent strains of the virus. This is a matter of confusion among the men of the AIDS Generation, and to this day, this issue of HIV reinfection remains hotly contested, with no clear definitive evidence that microbiological manifestations of reinfection manifest clinically. This controversy is clearly demonstrated in this posting from 1999 by David Salyer on the HIV information website, http://www.thebody.com:

> From virtually the beginning of this epidemic, there seemed to be a unanimous opinion that HIV-positive individuals could be reinfected by other strains of the virus. Two years ago, Dr. Branson told a roomful of HIV counselors that to date no evidence existed to support the theory of reinfection. He further stated his personal belief, not sanctioned by the CDC, that reinfection does not occur. I was not the only person in that room who bristled. This was radical stuff. And from that day forward I would hear his name and think, "Oh, yeah...that heretic guy from the CDC...I wonder when they'll fire him?"...Dr. David Ho, esteemed AIDS researcher, was quoted in Treatment News magazine saying, "There is little evidence to document that additional superinfection or reinfection with a second strain of HIV occurs at a period of time after infection." Jay Levy, an AIDS researcher at the University of California at San Francisco, states in his article in *HIV and the Pathogenesis of AIDS* that "in the host, resistance to superinfection appears to occur once the immune system has responded (or after seroconversion). Coinfection between individuals with HIV appears to be an uncommon event." Levy further acknowledges that "the prevalence of infection by more than one strain of HIV-1 in vivo (the body) is unknown but is most probably rare."...What have we learned? Reinfection research is inconclusive for now. Uncommon. Rare. Little evidence. Unknown. Not exactly the words most of us are looking for here.

It is within this swirling mass of inconsistent opinions that some of the men of the AIDS Generation came to make their decisions about their sexual behaviors to protect both their own physical well-being and that of their sexual and/or romantic partners. Answers were not simple and resulted in many attempts like my own "Ask the Sexpert" column in *Poz*, a periodical addressing the needs of the seropositive community; Kerry's advice column in *A&U* (described later in the chapter); and books such as *Love in the Time of HIV: A Gay Men's Guide to Sex, Dating, and Relationships* (2003), in which Michael Mancilla and Lisa Troshinsky provide hackneyed advice: "The virus doesn't have to mean an end to love and romance."

Antoine's approach to his physical health is illustrative of the management of risk behaviors. In this section of our discussion, Antoine indicates he attended to both his sexual health and that of his partners and did not rely on the use of substances:

PERRY: And you were taking care of yourself. Like you weren't drugging. You weren't really drinking. Pot is medicinal, so it's fine.

ANTOINE: Right.

PERRY: It's not having an immuno-compromising effect.

ANTOINE: I mean—and I was still having sex—

PERRY: Of course.

ANTOINE: —but I was using condoms.

PERRY: You were using condoms?

ANTOINE: Yeah.

PERRY: From the time you tested positive?

ANTOINE: Yeah. Because I felt ashamed that I would give this to somebody else.

PERRY: Even when you were bottoming?

ANTOINE: Yeah. Oh yeah.

PERRY: You would disclose? Or would you just insist on condoms?

ANTOINE: No because it was basically one-night stands, so I felt you didn't need to know.

PERRY: So they just, you just insisted that they use condoms, topping or bottoming?

ANTOINE: Yeah.

For some of the men of the AIDS Generation, the decision for safer sex was clear. In this regard, Hal, who, despite his outward appearance of steaming sultriness steeped in sexual tension, articulated his approach to his physical health and sex as follows: "I would never have sex with—I had believed when I'd stopped having unsafe sex that if I were to reinfect myself it'd increase the chances of me dying." He further describes it as follows:

> When safe sex and safer sex was discovered, when we knew the mode of transmission, I would say safe sex is like low-tar cigarettes. You smoke more of them, which takes you to how I took care of myself.

Yet for Gianni, the approach was to not spread the infection, but it was also reflective of the confusion around reinfection: "I made a commitment to sex with only positive men but not necessarily to safer sex with my poz partners." Still, he too was directed by his own physical health in his decision making: "Anyway I think neg guys might be carrying stuff they don't know about and give it to me. Poz guys are seeing a doctor all the time." This idea presented by Gianni was borne out in our previous research that had shown that gay HIV-positive men who engaged in unprotected sex with other HIV-positive men have a decreased belief that infection with other pathogens or reinfection with HIV presents a health problem (Halkitis, Green, et al., 2005), a situation also present in the context of primary relationships (Halkitis, Wilton, Parsons, & Hoff, 2004).

Sex has always been central to Jackson's life experiences: "I tended— I think while I liked to have sex, and I liked to have a lot of sex, and I did trick, and some of those experiences were delightful." Within the backdrop of safer sex and after his diagnosis, Jackson's overall approach to sex became directed toward his physical health and part of his overall holistic approach to health and well-being that included safe sex, health, and diet:

> And I became very careful. You know, once they knew what safe sex was, you know, I became very careful. There were a combination—if—if I could plug as many leaks as I could in terms of the information, in terms of my approach to health and diet and exercise—you know, all that was good. I had—I never—I had—I was curious about drugs, and so I tried them all. But I didn't have—and alcohol. I didn't—I never had a real trigger for them. So I didn't cave in.

One other point with regard to the realignment of sex as a means of improving physical health must be made. For three of the men with whom I spoke, Gianni, Ryan, and Christopher, there was not an abundant and extravagant sexual life prior to contracting the virus. Gianni, in fact, traces his seroconversion to his second sexual encounter with a man at age 18:

> So I—I'm pretty sure I knew that I was positive since, uh, the early '80s, and the reason why I thought that was because a man who I had been with, who is actually the second man who I'd ever had sex with when I was 18 years old, um, got sick and ended up dying in 8—1985. So, um, I was pretty sure that I was positive at that point when he died. And when he got diagnosed with, um, lymphoma a year before he died. But I didn't know for sure that I was positive, like with a test. Um, well I couldn't know in 1985 'cause there was no test.

For Ryan and Christopher, the youngest of the men I interviewed, sexual life was limited and informed by safe sex strategies, making their seroconversion even more surprising, given that both were engaging in the practices that should have kept them safe and both seroconverted in 1991, when information was more abundant than was the case for Gianni. Christopher described finding out about his status as follows:

> And that was really significant for me because I—I could count—when I found out I had HIV, I could count the number of people I was with on almost one hand, not quite. And I remember telling Douglas [a former befriend].... Um, I remember it was the only—at—to that—to that point, it was the only, um, anonymous encounter I ever had.

These stories illustrate the point that all it takes is once instance to seroconvert. And for these three young men, this one instance occurred early in their young adulthood when their sex lives were only beginning to emerge. Thus, there was no need to realign their approach to sex. They had not developed full repertoires of their sexual behaviors, and from that point forward, HIV would inform how they approached this aspect of their lives.

Overcoming Addiction

As with sexual behaviors, care of the physical self also took the form of actions to address the use of alcohol and other drugs. For Ryan, Christopher, and Kerry, substance use was not part of their narrative. For several of the men, like John, Bobby, Andre, Tyronne, and Eddie, these behaviors preceded the AIDS epidemic, and realignment toward drugs emerged over a period of time. For Ralph, substance use was clearly the result of living in a world of death caused by AIDS. However, for one of the men, Hal, actions were swift and immediate.

In the case of Hal, the voice of sobriety was powerful and permeated much of our conversation. For Hal, this self-care took the form of addressing his substance use first and foremost: "I had a history of substance abuse and when I was diagnosed I stopped doing drugs, drinking."

However, for most of the men who had relied on substances over the course of their lives, such as John, Bobby, Andre, Tyronne, and Eddie, sobriety did not emerge immediately after diagnosis but rather over the course of time. This relationship toward substances was only modified when it became clear to each of them that reliance on substances was compromising their physical well-being, usually after reaching "rock bottom." These stories are examined later in the chapter (in the section The Power of Escape).

For all of the men of the AIDS Generation, regardless of when these potentially harmful behavioral patterns were terminated, controlling their substance use and sexual lives was a means of enhancing and protecting physical health, but these actions also improved and heightened their emotional and social well-being.

The Emotional Self

The behavioral research literature indicates that the management of emotional well-being is critical in the well-being of HIV-positive individuals. It is posited that emotional disclosure and the management of stressors have a beneficial effect on the immune systems of HIV-positive individuals (Bower, Kemeny, Taylor, & Fahey, 1998; O'Cleirigh, Ironson, Fletcher, & Schneiderman, 2008). This ability to process emotions and release emotional burdens has been related to a variety of positive health outcomes including long-term survival in people living with HIV (O'Cleirigh et al., 2003). These findings complement the work of Barroso (1997; Barroso, Buchanan, Tomlinson, & Van Servellen, 1997), which indicates that taking care of oneself is critical to surviving AIDS, and care for self includes decreasing stress and discontinuing negative habits. Such an approach to surviving AIDS and caring for his well-being is evident in Hal's life in 1987, a few years after his diagnosis in Connecticut:

> Um, it became really clear to me that I could not use drugs. It just became, like, crystal clear one day. I was snorting coke up a bloody nose and

I thought, "This is—something's wrong here." So I sought treatment. And then in treatment developed sort of a will to live, desire to live.

The ability to manage negative emotional states is critical to the well-being of HIV-positive men. In her program of research, Jane Leserman (2003) showed that depression, stress, and trauma have negative effects on the emotional well-being of seropositive individuals—states that also impact physical well-being. Thus, the management of these conditions is critical to the lives of those living with HIV. In Chapter 3, I commented on the role of trauma and the management of this condition postdiagnosis, in what I referred to as "the pause." Here, I consider the variety of strategies the men utilized to mange their emotional well-being.

Hal quickly reduced his reliance on substances and sought social support through the community-developed networks. Others, as will be noted, engaged in the therapeutic process to release emotional burdens, whereas others derived this enhancement of the emotional life through the love relationships they developed.

Releasing Emotional Burdens

Emotional self-care also requires a release of emotional burdens. One manner to understand care for emotional well-being is through a model of cognitive processing, a way of knowing that includes awareness, perception, and reasoning. This type of cognition has been associated with better health outcomes following stressful events (e.g., Pennebaker, Kiecolt-Glaser, & Glaser, 1988). Specifically as it relates to HIV, cognitive processing of life events may be critical in maintenance of both emotional and physical health: "The process of thinking about a stressful event may lead to a number of different psychological outcomes, such as regaining a sense of mastery over one's life or regaining one's self-esteem" (Bower et al., 1998, p. 979). This is how Eddie has come to understand his survival, by attending to his emotions, accepting his sexuality and his disease, and expressing his ideas and emotions as a mentor to at-risk young gay men:

> I think what sort of sustained me is my attitude about just believing that I'm healthy and I'm okay regardless of what's going on with my body really helped me. I didn't really feel or allow this disease to sort of inhibit how I sort of looked or viewed life at all. I was in denial with my own sexuality, with just sort of being able to disclose openly to everyone. I think a big part of my survival has been coming to grips with accepting who I am, being

proud of who I am. I am a mentor; I am an example for I think the gay community in general.

For Ryan, there was a need to take proactive steps to contain his emotional well-being and to deter the psychological burdens he was experiencing due to his seropositive status. Ryan, who at age 40 is now married to his love of some 20 years, Zack, took a multipronged approach to keeping his emotional well-being intact, including allowing his emotions to be expressed and seeking support from others who were also HIV positive:

> I lost it sometimes. I was extremely fearful of every rash, sneeze, scratch, or anything at the beginning. I read a lot—probably too much—about symptoms of OIs [opportunistic infections] and drove myself crazy over what always turned out to be very normal things for someone HIV-negative or HIV positive. Also, I went for group therapy at GMHC, which gave me a small community of folks who I knew, understood my issues.

Moreover, when he reached age 30 as an HIV-positive man, the mixture of emotional states required further support that he quickly sought. Ryan was keenly in tune with his emotional well-being and undertook approaches to care to ensure that these burdens would not compromise his overall life and would allow him to proceed into living:

> At 30, though, I went into a depression and began individual therapy. At that point I also began antidepressants and am still on them to this day. I think the mark of 30 was something so unexpected and for some reason instead of just being happy, threw my emotions into a frenzy.

So, too, Hal spoke of his strategy to manage his emotions in light of the ongoing demands of living with HIV. It is clear that when Hal speaks of this aspect of his life, the management of these emotional states is one that he consciously considers and recognizes in himself and his HIV-positive friends:

> I also—I have a lot of HIV—well not a lot, I've got four HIV-positive friends who've been—who've had AIDS or have been positive as long as I have. For like 28 years or slightly more. And while we all manage our illnesses a little differently emotionally, the nuts and bolts of everyday care or taking our meds, all that kind of stuff, tend to engender the same kind of emotional response and also it's pretty similar.

Hal, whose zeal is illustrative of his passionate nature, elaborated on this idea, indicating how emotional release has been critical to his survival, and a behavior that was not reflected in his upbringing and he had to learn. Such emotional responses might have seemed contradictory to anyone who saw Hal, a very masculine, somewhat hypermasculine, extremely fit man, who on the surface might appear to have never shed a tear in his life:

> I was thrown into intramural sports at the age of 4 and I played them until 12th grade. I had brothers who constantly were picking physical fights with me. I was raised to push back and to fight and to be strong and to—when my mother died it was, "Be strong." I mean to some of a detriment because there were emotions that I later expressed that were bottled up and—oh that's another thing that I really, really, truly, ultimately believe that saved my life. That at a certain point I learned how to express my feelings and I never stopped. I cry when I'm sad. I cry when I—I get choked up when I talk about my husband. I laugh my ass off. I have the entire range of feelings appropriately but I have them strongly. And I think by not releasing those feelings—you were setting yourself up for disease.

The Love of a Good Man (as First Noted by Michael Callen [1990])

Taking care of one's emotional self also was realized in the loving relationships some of the men forged. This was particularly true for two of the men of the AIDS Generation, Ryan and Christopher. Recall that both men are the youngest of the AIDS Generation cohort with whom I spoke, 40 and 45, respectively, and both were diagnosed in 1991 despite their "safe sex" strategies to that point. Interestingly, at the time of diagnosis both also had embarked on new relationships, relationships that are sustained to this day, and relationships with men who were and continue to be HIV-negative. Thus, safer sex within the context of a loving relationship had power and meaning for both men, which required careful negotiation and balancing of both their sexual behaviors and their emotions with regard to sex. In this regard both succeeded.

Both Ryan and Christopher expressed how their attention to preventing their partners from becoming infected held significant meaning. It would be easy to say that this strategy was directed toward the physical health of their partners, but it is clear that these decisions and actions were ultimately driven by protecting their own emotional lives, which were fragile at the time of diagnosis. In this regard, Christopher described these challenges in his relationship with his partner Bruce as follows:

> It was really hard to do. Um, we sort of took the lowest common denominator, you know. Like what was—I think what was safe to him and what was safe to me might have been two different things, so we always took the—the greater precaution, if you will. So oral sex was always with condoms. You know, which I hated. Um, and we didn't really have a lot of—we had a little bit of anal sex, but we didn't have a ton of it because he always had issues with hemorrhoids and this kind of thing. So that was never like a big thing. And I probably—it's probably good because he probably would have it because there were a ton of times, you know, like we had oral sex unprotected in the first year [before seroconversion]. But I can remember and I don't think he ever swallowed.

The action toward safer sex described by Christopher certainly protected his partner's health but also provided a level of protection for himself. Although Christopher did not articulate this strategy as a means of protecting his physical health, it was clear that the strategy provided a level of emotional protection, insomuch as he was caring for his partner and would not carry the burden of infecting him with HIV. Ryan and his now husband Zack also approached the decision to engage in safer sex with love and respect for each other.In fact, Ryan's now husband was very emotionally supportive as Ryan navigated the difficult early days of his seroconversion:

> Um, he had a, he had an easier time with it than I did. Um, he kind of took things as they came, and I think that came with just his experience, you know, most recently. And I was the one who was kind of the neurotic, you know, which is, you know. Not unlikely anyway. But you know, kind of the, you know, the neurotic, um, you know—I mean, this was, you know, besides being positive, this was also my first serious relationship. I mean, I was—yeah. I mean, if it's, you know—we moved in together a few months later. Um, like early '92. Um, so it was a, a lot was going on. Being in a relationship, and then positive on top of all of that.

From both these narratives, it is clear that both partners of Ryan and Christopher and their respective relationships played a significant part in protecting the well-being of the men whom they loved and continue to love. Both had just embarked on a new relationship at the time their partners were diagnosed, both are still in a relationship with these men, and both clearly provided emotional support to Ryan and Christopher. Eaton, West, Kenny, and Kalichman (2009) have shown that partners are a significant source of influence, and Remien, Wagner, Dolezal, and Carballo-Dieguez (2002) have shown that both biological and behavioral factors influence the decision making of these couples. These elements appear in the narratives of Ryan and Christopher, and above all what appears more clearly in the narratives is the love a good man who was caring for the emotional life of his partner, who had just received a life-ending diagnosis. This is not to say that neither of their partners was self-protecting from HIV, as is often the case in gay male couples (Appleby, Miller, & Rothspan, 1999), but the emotional care of their HIV-infected partners was also front and center. So, for both Ryan and Christopher, maintaining a viable, vibrant, and healthy relationship was a powerful and effective emotional strategy to handle their diagnoses and allowed them to move forward with their lives and into the world.

Emotional support in the context of the relationship permeates the lives of both men to this day, although the dynamics have changed. In the case of Christopher, time has taken its toll on their sexual life, as it does for many couples. Yet what is clear is that the relationship and emotional support he receives from the man he loves is as significant to this day as it was 20 years ago, even in the absence of sex:

> We're not having sex together. There's affection there. I kiss him good-bye every morning. Um, I spoon with him. We do a lot of stuff together. We also do stuff apart.

Ryan told a similar story. Still, Ryan describes this emotional support that certainly involved his husband but also extends to others in his family. When I asked him what keeps him alive and what sustained him even before the advent of active retroviral therapy (ART) in 1996, Ryan said: "Um, I think over time different things have pushed me towards that. Um, I would say, you know, early on through now, it's definitely been my husband."

Finally, in the case of Kerry, who during our interview spoke often of the need to bring together the community of HIV-positive men, the love a good man only emerged in the last few years. Yet, like Ryan and Christopher, the relationship provides him with emotional fortitude that is illustrative of this strategy that some men of the AIDS Generation have used and still use to survive. But perhaps Kerry's desire for self-care in his social life was most evident as he spoke of his partner and the home life they have created together. It is when he spoke of this relationship that Kerry was most radiant and seemed fulfilled. It was clear both in his words and in his smile that this relationship is one that provides him with the strength to manage his HIV disease:

Um, he works. Uh, sometimes I work that nonjob. I'm home. He comes home; he's got a really fucked-up schedule. We're never in the same place at the same time. . . . I mean like he's a—he's a funny little guy, he's a character. So he's, um, he's older in a lot of ways. He'll sit and make bowties while I'm on Facebook. He'll make bowties out of his old vintage ties to save money—um, while I'm on Facebook yapping about some drag show. That's pretty much it—it sounds crazy. . . . He makes dinner. I clean up. He, um, usually goes in the—he smokes and I make him smoke by a window in the bedroom and he does it all the time. And then he'll watch Discovery Channel in one room and I'll watch what I want in the other room. And then we meet in bed at night.

The Social Self

Attendance to the social self was yet another strategy many of the men of the AIDS Generation enacted to attend to self-care. Either through support groups, through their involvement in community and activist organizations, or simply by immersing themselves with others who were facing the same conditions, the men of the AIDS Generation built their social capital, which ameliorated isolation and enhanced overall health.

The social determinants of health and well-being are an area of particular importance in the domain of public health and have garnered much attention in the last two decades. In this perspective, health is driven by numerous factors that extend beyond simple behavior. As is the view in an ecosocial paradigm, health is directed by individual-level factors but also social and environmental factors (Krieger, 2001). The Centers for Disease Control and Prevention (CDC) recently espoused such an understanding, recognizing that a holistic approach to health and well-being requires that we attend to social determinants, including social networks and social support, the neighborhood in which we live, and the environments we navigate, as well as social and economic systems (CDC, 2010). Kapadia et al. (2013) consider the role that social cohesion and social support play in understanding the well-being of gay men and the manner in which engagement in such social networks may provide protective effects.

This is all to say that the social well-being of HIV-positive men is critical—a condition that the men of the AIDS Generation recognized long before there was an abundant academic literature to support the importance of social well-being. ACT UP and GMHC are but two examples of the social structures we built. As members of these organizations, we fought for the development of and access to treatment and provided care for those who were ailing, but mostly we created entities that provided social cohesion and social support. There is a rich and abundant literature from the pre-ART era on the role of social systems and HIV disease progression, providing evidence of social support as a protective factor (e.g., Solano et al., 1993; Theorell et al., 1995).

Being in relation to others is a dimension that has been related to survival among the HIV positive, especially in the pre-ART era (Barroso, 1997). Such social connectedness helped to enhance the ability of the men of the AIDS Generation to confront their disease and face the challenges head on—what I will describe later in this chapter as "the spirit." Moreover, these social systems, in the form of community-building activism and love relationships, were significant in the life stories of the men of the AIDS Generation. For Hal, such structures were key to his survival: "So I've always—I've been in three support groups, one at GMHC in the beginning and then two in Provincetown, one lasting 5 years and one lasting 7 years."

Combating Isolation and Building Social Capital

The voice of the social self and of its associated care was most pronounced in the interview with Kerry. In both our interactions, one on one and in the focus group, Kerry expressed concern about his social well-being and the problems that he faced in terms of his career and his place in the world. Much of his effort for self-care was thus directed toward making meaning of his life and ensuring the social fabric of his life. It was clear that this desire was a form of self-care, even before he was diagnosed with HIV:

And, um, I remember maybe '82 or '83 Gay Pride, before I was even positive, handing out condoms because of my lover and people like kind of scoffing at me. And I saw it happen again recently where—oh, I know—it was the Folsom East thing, and go through like hell with the drugs and the drug trials. So I started handing out condoms. What's, like, my reaction was I'm gonna keep other people from getting this. I wouldn't want anyone to feel the way I did that day, or have to go through what I'm gonna have to go through.

It is clear in this statement that Kerry's actions are directed at a social good and his role as an agent of social change, which empowered him in the management of the disease even prior to his own infection. Similarly, he continued along this path after his infection, writing an advice column for other HIV-positive gay men:

> For 7 years I wrote an advice column for *A&U Magazine*… And that was cathartic for me too.…My activism mostly was in my column—and that was just people's—it was like a "Dear Abby" for people with AIDS.

Kerry's narrative also indicates that care of others was a form of care for his social self, which was evident in his volunteer efforts with a local AIDS service organization, even before he was infected:

> I did volunteer work. Like we cleaned out rooms of—with the—I forget what AIDS—see, that's the other thing. My memory's not great. The AIDS organization used to go and clean out houses and then put somebody in—and then they'd die, and then you'd go clean it, and then they'd put somebody in and someone else would die and you'd go clean it and put somebody in.

Jackson articulates and situates his strategies to enhance the social self as highly activist, a self-perception, label, and identity he carries to this day. As part of the theater community in New York City, Jackson experienced much loss early in the epidemic, which provided him the impetus to be involved, to work on behalf of his community, and ultimately to work on behalf of himself. It may seem odd to the reader that I situate these activists and volunteering activities as self-serving and as a means for understanding care for the social self. In the 30 years since the onset of AIDS, the collective narrative we have developed portrays the formation of these social agencies such as ACT UP as altruistic and working toward the good for all. I do not dispute that fact. However, it was our own individual desires to live and self-care that brought us together. We were all individually at risk, and our own personal struggles and need to self-care bonded us to create these organizations and these movements. It was not an amorphous ideal—there was an actual need we each had and we came together to provide it to each other, in the same manner that immigrants flock to similar neighborhoods, creating ghettos. These collectives provide social support and cohesion and a buffer against isolation, loneliness, and potential despair. I remember this thought also as I watched the

Oscar-nominated documentary of ACT UP, *How to Survive a Plague*. I turned to my husband Bobby during the first screening in New York and whispered, "These guys simply wanted to live and they found each other. We all found each other." Jackson further articulates this idea of activism as social cohesion. After a period of 6 months "turning off" after his diagnosis, Jackson reemerged into his social milieu, which provided him with the support to further care for himself:

> Yeah. I just, uh—I had to think....Then it turned into being in ACT UP, reading these treatment data, trying to get as much information as I possibly could out of that, you know, and finding the tools and listen and watching people die and seeing, you know—it's hard to figure out what they did. And seeing the example of people in ACT UP, Peter Staley included, who could stand up and say I'm HIV positive and seeing these tough, strong, you know, fighters and—and drawing strength from them.

This social cohesion, with ACT UP, also provided Jackson the strength to face his own possible mortality:

> But I did—I had thrown myself into the AIDS crisis as an activist already and I think it bumped it up in terms of reading the treatment and data information and, and, going to as many memorial services. And I got really good at delivering eulogies and I would really throw myself in and, when I joined ACT UP, I thought well I'm just being an altruistic good guy. And I realized in hindsight, I think I was picking up tools and, you know, seeing survival because I remember watching someone take their last breath, demystifying death for me and making me less afraid of it all.

I think many of us who were living in the midst of the crisis sought the solace, and activism, in whatever form we could. For Robert it was being the first editor of *The Body Positive*, a periodical replete with helpful information that emerged from the now-defunct AIDS service organization of the same name. For Peter Staley and Mark Harrington and the other protagonists of *How to Survive a Plague,* it was ACT UP and the Treatment Action Group (TAG). For Ryan and Hal, it was working and being clients at GMHC. In whatever form, these organizations and institutions brought us together, lessened our isolation, and enhanced our social capital.

For the last several decades, the public health literature has provided ample evidence for the protective effects of social capital on health outcomes (Krieger, 2001; Link & Phelan, 1995; Whitehead & Diderichsen,

2001), including HIV (Poundstone, Strathdee, & Celentano, 2004). Using a psychological framework in the Sacramento Health Study enacted prior to widespread implementation of ART, Herek and Glunt (1995) showed that community involvement is critical for alleviating feelings of depression and enhancing self-esteem in gay men who were on average in their early 30s in the early 1990s—that is, the men of the AIDS Generation. Through these volunteer and activist institutions, the social capital of the AIDS Generation provided protection from the ravaging effects of HIV. These protective effects of social capital are evident in the epidemic to this day, and lack thereof explains heightened rates of disease in the Black population of the United States (Cené et al., 2011).

In speaking with Jackson, it became clear that his approach to self-care through the social contexts he navigated and through his involvement with ACT UP was his means of controlling the virus. By engaging in these institutions he remained abreast of the latest knowledge, and with this knowledge came an underlying belief that he could handle the disease intellectually, that he could outsmart it. Jackson describes this notion of power as knowledge as he clearly recalled first reading one of the accounts of AIDS in *The New York Times* with his friends: "We scoured it sentence by sentence looking for clues and, you know, going with the purple spots and how much they had set. I mean, everything we did." After the conclusion of my interview with Jackson, I reflected as follows:

> Jackson, 57 years old, White, blue eyes, wore a polo shirt—a shirt buttoned up really high and jeans. Um, beautiful white hair, very handsome. The power of his story, um, and the center of his story is sort of focused on and centered on, um, thoughtfulness around HIV and mind over matter. How he managed the disease by learning and knowing and thinking and plotting. And it's sort of like [a] methodical approach to the disease, and almost like a methodical approach to life. Everything was very circumspect and very, like, planned out. And I think that's how he's managed it, and that's how he's managed his life.

Immersion With Others Like Me

The attention to social well-being also emerged in the story of Ralph, but in a somewhat different manner. Ralph was born and raised in Salt Lake City, which he described as a somewhat small town, made even smaller when the AIDS epidemic emerged. So, when he and his partner Colin discovered that they had been infected with HIV, their actions were swift and immediate—a relocation to San Francisco to be among others who were experiencing the same conditions: "I had a partner at the time and, you know, we both tested positive and so we decided being in Utah wasn't really the place to be so we went to San Francisco together." The small-town mentality of Salt Lake City, coupled with the stigmatized view of HIV, necessitated this move:

> Oh, I remember. It was, um, I mean, it was all new at the time and, um, I remember people, um, that, you know—there was gossip about people that had tested positive or that had, um, you know, HIV/AIDS or whatever it was called then; I don't really remember, and um, I had had sex with one of the people that everybody was gossiping about.

Despite a time of little hope, the move to San Francisco appeared to be the best option for Ralph and Colin to be among others who were also living with the disease, to have access to the best care, and to not feel stigmatized and isolated. Their move to San Francisco was driven by many factors, but the one that Ralph most clearly voiced was that of care for the social self. Living with HIV in Utah would have simply been too difficult: "Um, but we also were thinking let's, um, get together with more of our kind because we don't want to be outcasts in a horrible city where—let's get together with—you know, it was like a corral, let's get into the corral...."

Like many of the men of the AIDS Generation, there was desire on Ralph's part to ameliorate the feelings of stigma, to create a greater sense of social cohesion, and to address through social engagement the feelings of loneliness and desperation often associated with those who were living with AIDS. Cities like San Francisco and New York provided such contexts, as did the many wonderful community-based organizations and initiatives, such as GMHC, that emerged at the time. These community connections were critical to our survival, as noted by Remien and Rabkin (1995), and volunteerism in such organizations enhanced social networks and connections (Omoto & Crain, 1995). Drawing data from interviews conducted at GMHC in 1990, Remien and Rabkin (1995, p. 169) note the critical role that the HIV community and AIDS service organizations played in "...maintaining the person's conviction that life has value despite progressive illness."

The need to be with others "like me" is as true today for the men of the AIDS Generation as it was early in their diagnosis. When the men gathered for the focus group, the bond was immediate and tangible. In the midst of the conversation, Kerry verbalized the meaning of being with others who have lived and continue to live with the conditions of HIV:

> The horror. The horrible stuff. The horrible stuff that we all lived through. And until he said that [Hal describing the losses to AIDS], it didn't really dawn on me. But you can't really forget about that stuff either because that's like he said. You didn't have a choice; when you want to live, you want to live. That's it. You do what you have to. But it's funny that he should say it seemed like it never happened because in some ways, it seemed like it never happened.
>
> And something like this [focus group] makes, gets me choked up because I think oh thank God, there's other people who are there, who saw it, who know it, who lived through it because we're few and far between. [Eddie: "Absolutely."] I don't recognize—I expected to come here and recognize everyone who was here. [Hal: "I thought the same thing."] But I don't know anybody here, which to me is another odd thing. I just figured we'd be whittled down to the same people we see all the time. And it's a comfort to know that there's so many of us still around.

To this point, Hal also commented on the comfort of simply knowing others are present even through nonverbal connections:

> Well, it's funny too from this side effects we're experiencing from treatment, like I've had filler in my face and other things done. But it's um—I spot us. Every now and then I'll walk by and go—I'll see a 50- to 60-year-old and go, yeah, I know what that is. I know why he looks that way.

In a time of little hope, this social connection with others who were waging the same war lessened the blow of the AIDS epidemic. It still is a connection that the men of the AIDS Generation desire and need, as evidenced in the strong bonds the men formed while participating in the focus group.

The Will to Live and Face Death Head On (aka "the Spirit")

As has been shown, across all the men of the AIDS Generation, there was no defined approach or set of approaches to the management of their disease. Although all recognized the need to attend to their whole person, each spoke of varying strategies for addressing their physical, emotional, and social well-being. Consistently, however, they all voiced one common element—the will to survive and face their disease even when the probability for survival was minimal at best. This is perhaps why the men developed the multitude of strategies to cope with their illness. Underlying these approaches was a belief that one would survive and a belief that one could confront and defeat HIV. None of the men voiced a sense of defeat even in their darkest moments. To this point, Ralph indicated, "I think there's a survival, I mean, drawing a breath is a choice. You choose to live every time you draw a breath." Hal voiced this approach to the disease eloquently:

> I've always considered myself someone who runs into a fire to save the baby and as far as AIDS and HIV have been concerned, I've run to it rather than away from it. But when it comes to crises or stresses I have a very strong lack of fear. I just—when those situations happen I don't know if it's an adrenalin response, I don't know exactly, I'm sure it's a biochemical thing that happens.

And for Gianni, who tested only after falling in love for the very first time, the will to live and continue on his life path was how he described his approach to his diagnosis: "I was just going. I knew what I wanted to do. It was like I kept moving. I kept moving. I kept moving as if nothing was going on." This will to fight the virus and continue on life's journey has followed men throughout the course of their lives as they keep on fighting off the ravages of HIV and the new attacks that emerge on the body, mind, and spirit. Richard, whose musical about surviving AIDS has been performed around the world, voiced this will even after a bout of recent illness:

> I have an indomitable spirit, I believe. And just a need to live, but lately I've been attacked on all fronts by a lot of different things. A couple of months ago I got a kidney stone and then I got another one last week. And I feel as weak as a kitten right now. And I'm starting to feel like an old tire that keeps getting repumped up and still has holes in it. And I was feeling that way walking around today that I just can't seem to get back on top with the spirit that I had been before. And I'll get through this; I believe that I'll get through this.

For Antoine, his spirit was never broken, despite the loss of almost his entire social circle. Instead, these life experiences built his spirit and his resolve to live. His life as an HIV-positive man has helped him develop a fortitude he would not have developed had he had not seroconverted and had he not been gay. Like many of the men of the AIDS Generation, this power, fortitude, and spirit to go on despite all odds was developed through living a life of ongoing struggles negotiating sexuality in a hetero-normative society. For many, HIV was just another struggle, as expressed in the words of Antoine:

> Even though I've lost a lot of dear, dear friends… It was a learning experience. And each one, I learned something different about me, that I can be residual. I can be forceful. I can be determined, and I'm a good fighter. And I'm going to be in it for the long haul.

This, too, was the case for Eddie. Despite a long and complicated foray into substance use that took him from Detroit, to Atlanta, back to Detroit, then to Los Angeles, and eventually to New York City, his beliefs about his survival dominated his handling of HIV. He described it in the focus group as follows:

> So it was, to me, um, never—I never really felt like I was ever going to die. I never felt like I was really sick. And I've been really sick. I've been in the hospital, um, I lost the use of my left arm and my right leg completely. They wouldn't move. And it was due to the fact I had all this stuff going on. I forget what they call it. I can't think right now. Yeah, it was horrible. I was in a wheelchair and um, and a lot of it was just—and even in the hospital I was so sick, I never, ever thought I was gonna die. I think what sort of sustained me is my attitude about just believing that I'm healthy and I'm okay regardless of what's going on with my body really helped me. I didn't really feel or allow this disease to sort of inhibit how I sort of looked [at] or viewed life at all.

This overriding desire to live and make the most out of one's life also was apparent in the interviews with the men from Project Gold: "I was starting to have those first inclinations that I wanted to live. You know, life was worth fighting for." For another Project Gold participant, a 51-year-old Latin man, the desire to survive was intimately tied to his self- care:

> I learned to appreciate life a lot more. I learned to appreciate my family, my friends, my partners a lot more. Ah, that when I was in my 20s; life just

means a whole lot more now than it did back then. Ah, because I treasure life. I take care of myself a lot better. After being sick a few times in and getting very close to dying, it made me realize that if I don't take care of myself, I won't be around for long. That I have to really take very good care of myself.

The voices of these men perfectly demonstrate the attitudes toward life so many men of the AIDS Generation espoused in managing and negotiating their HIV diagnoses, as indicated by Patrick: "I think if I were pessimistic about it, it would be a different story. I've always had a positive attitude." And despite fearing death, a desire to live and keep moving was evident in Kerry's story in relation to AIDS:

Oh, it was so frightening. It was—I—I always kept, like, a distance from it though. I kind of, like, um, removed myself from it, like people say they have that bright light when they die, I always—as—as soon as I found out I pulled myself back and I thought I wanted to learn, I wanted to take it all in. Maybe I didn't think I had limited time because there was something about just taking it all in. I just wanted to experience everything. Because I figured by 35 I wouldn't be there anymore. And I'm still kind of, like, taking it all in. That's the best advice I've ever had for myself, was just, like, just enjoy the ride.

So, too, Patrick articulated a sensibility and will to survive and face the disease head on, and not be defined solely by his diagnosis:

There's other times, that came—this was just "How am I going to deal with this today? How am I going to be okay with this so that I can still be—at least present the happy face to the people I see and not be this 'Oh, my god, I've got AIDS'?" You know? I didn't want to be that person.

For Patrick, this attitude defined his outcomes and explains why he is still alive today. It is clear that for all of the men of the AIDS Generation with whom I spoke, there was an undeniable survival instinct. It is possible that this will to survive and this desire to live helped them actively confront and manage their disease. However, it would be shortsighted on my part to suggest that those of my generation who did not survive somehow were less proactive in their approach to the disease. To this point, the will to live is not a sufficient cause for explaining one's survival, but it is a necessary component. Clearly a set of physical, emotional, and social strategies contributed to this outcome for the men with whom I spoke. All strategies, including the will and spirit, are necessary. For some men, like Christopher, this state was understood in terms of proceeding with the course of life and not making any radical changes, rather than in terms of spirit, although it can be argued that these are overlapping ideas:

> I think for me it was just like I sort of stayed on a track and I'm like, "All right. Pretend I'm gonna live forever. And just do what you were gonna do and if it's cut short, it's cut short." So because I—I—I heard about people that just like sort of like quit their jobs or did like drastic things. And I was first of all never the kind of person that would do something like that—even if I didn't have HIV. And I would hear about these people that would do drastic things and it just never seemed to work out for them or—right, yeah, I sort of stayed the course.

In Chapter 1, I described the sufficient-component model of understanding disease (Aschengrau & Seage, 2008). I draw from this theory again to describe causal pathways to survival among the men of the AIDS Generation. It is clear that one set of strategies alone or attention to only one domain of existence cannot suffice in leading to this outcome. The men with whom I spoke indicated attention to the whole, and the whole consisted of the physical, the emotional, and the social. To that mix of necessary but individually insufficient components I add one more domain—the spiritual.

I have come to understand the will to survive as "the spirit." Along with the care to the body, to the mind, and to the social being, attention to the spirit has been a critical component in the strategies the men have developed over the course of their lives. I do not seek to attach a religious component to how I come to understand the spirit. Suffice it to say that in the lives of the men of the AIDS Generation, the instinct to survive—the indomitable will—is how I come to understand the spirit. And although it alone cannot ensure or guarantee the survival of the men to this day, it was a crucial and necessary element in their lives. In the behavioral literature, this construct has also been referred to as dispositional optimism and has been related to slower disease progression for HIV-positive individuals even before the implementations of ART in 1996 (Milam, Richardson, Marks, Kemper, & McCutchan, 2004; Ironson et al., 2005). Even after the implementation of ART, positive outlooks in the form of positive affect, finding meaning, and optimistic expectancy have been related to lower mortality and immune system decline (Ickovics et al., 2006). Moreover, such affective states have been linked to biological manifestations. Specifically, positive outlook has been shown to be related to lower levels of the stress hormones cortisol and norepinephrine, among others; these patterns suggest a casual pathway between positive outlook, hormones, and HIV-related health (Ironson & H'Sien, 2008).

To nurture the spirit and to develop such optimistic outlooks, it became essential for the men to define themselves beyond their HIV. The point is that these men chose to neither be defined solely by their virus nor defeated by HIV. Rather, they accepted their diagnoses but were not defined solely by their diagnoses. Such a form of coping, which suggests a healthy acceptance, has been related to the delay of AIDS-related complications in a study of gay and bisexual men (Reed, Kemeny, Taylor, Wang, & Visscher, 1994). Along these lines, Bobby, whose roots were laid in his youth in Louisiana, shared the following ideas:

> I—you talk about spirituality and I've always been—I had to break away from a Southern Baptist traditional upbringing. But I tricked with a Tai-Chi instructor in college and he taught me a move that's called "Embrace Tiger; Return to Mountain." It's a crazy trip but I still remember. It was one night but I still remember the philosophy: it was not to go out and attack a tiger or try to kill it, slay the dragon. The idea is to understand this beast and respect it and embrace it and return it safely to the mountain where it belongs. And I think that's been a driving philosophy.

However, of all the stories, Richard's story best exemplifies the power of the spirit and the ability to exist beyond the boundaries of HIV. For Richard, the spirit and the will to live helped him survive a very dark period of his life when all hope was lost. Richard describes being incredibly ill and how his illness forced him to abandon his music, which had been central to his identity, his life, and his livelihood. To help rebuild his spirit during this critical juncture in his life, Richard once again turned to his great love, his music. In this regard, Richard relied on his social circle, his social support system, to help him reimmerse into the world after a year-long battle with an extremely severe case of *Pneumocystis* pneumonia (PCP). And although the research on the benefits of social support on the well-being of those with HIV has yielded mixed findings, this factor has been related to better health outcomes in several studies, especially in those studies conducted prior to the widespread implementation of ART in the United States. In a study of 96 men conducted by Leserman et al. (1999, 2000, 2002), higher levels of social support were related to slower disease progression. It is in this period, pre-ART, that Richard relied on his social systems to reengage with his life:

> So now I'm—I'm spending this year—I was spending this solid year or more doing nothing but trying to build my body back up to, um, some semblance of functionality....And just trying to stay connected to the rest of the world from my hospital bed—I mean, from my—from my home.
>
> And then I—I did the same thing with a music publisher friend of mine. We were very close friends. And I said can I just—I'll sweep the floors if I could just have an excuse to get up and come to the office. And this was kind of a life-changing, um, moment for me because they—they were very aware of the work that I had done at National Academy of Song Writers. So on the first day that I showed up to just do anything, they actually had a desk for me, and they had business cards and a title. And they made me like the creative director. And they said you have great ears, and you know how to talk to young writers. And so we'll just bring all the young writers in, and you can talk to them and listen to music. And we'll give you an actual position. It wasn't a paid position because they didn't really have money. But the respect was very self-motivating and—and—and brings me to tears even to think about it. In July of 1995, I hadn't played much music. And I remember that my Aunt anny the one I had told you—she was living in Vegas. She called me and wanted to know how I was doing. And I didn't quite know how to put it into words. So, um, I got up to the piano—until then, I was too weak to sit up for—very much at all.

And as Richard reengaged with his music, he found that his spirit strengthened, having an impact on all aspects of his well-being beyond simply the physical, although that is what was most apparent to him:

> But I began to play music. And I—I remember this one—this very first day that I was doing it. I had a little upright, and I leaned my head up against the wood of the piano, and remember, for this past year, I've been trying very hard to build myself up. So I played all my favorite chords, or these big, rich, gospel kind of chords and just played and played and played for hours maybe. I don't know. It just went on. And the next day when I woke up, I felt normal. And that's when I knew that the vibrations of the music, the creating of music had a measurable, physical effect on my body.

When I asked Richard to describe what he meant by saying he felt normal, he indicated:

> Normal means I was probably up to about 85% of real normal. I didn't feel that persistent weakness that I had felt. There was always a sort of a weakness. I don't have another word for it. That was always lingering when I would walk across the room or do something.

Then Richard described with great detail and beauty the building of his spirit and the building of his body and his emotional well-being as he continued to craft his music:

> I no longer felt the sickness. I knew my body was sick. And I'm not saying this in a metaphysical sense. I mean that it felt like that I had risen up out of my sick body and was not observing it but just was in a state of unpain, of not pain by hearing that voice of love and hearing that voice of need. And I know that that was when I made the decision that I was going to survive. So I put that into a song. A song called "Connected." And when I finished writing this song, it took everything out of me. I was scribbling the words down so fast because they were coming to me whole.
>
> The whole song was coming to me absolutely word for word the way it ended up, except for a few minor changes because we always edit, right? And it exhausted me, and I—I even remember when I started to play the music for it, I played in a key that I don't play in, F sharp, which is all black keys, and it's difficult—and it's a difficult key. So I wrote the key in F sharp so that my fingers would not go anywhere that they normally are predisposed to go. And when I woke up the next day, I said to Phil [his partner], "I've written this song. I think I've written this song. I think it might be really good."
>
> Usually, I was very self-critical about my own music, and I didn't write hardly at all when I worked for National Academy of Song Writers. I was helping everybody else. So I sat down to play this song, and I got five words into it and began to ball like a baby. And every line, I would cry even more, and I would cry even more. And it finally got to the end of it. And, uh, Phil agreed with me that it was an extraordinary song. And so I started to go around and play it for my other songwriting friends, all of whom had long lists of credits, hit song writers, people who wrote for Michael Jackson, Madonna, all these other people.
>
> And whenever I would play that song for them, they would be thunderstruck. And Phil noticed as I sang that song and performed it for them that I would sit up straighter, breathe more easily, have more life in me. It

was making me stronger. Once again, that measurable, physical effect. So he started giving me ideas for more songs based on things that I had told him, like I went to a group therapy session. I went to, um, all the—all the fake cures that people were inundating me with, uh, a song about my own memorial service.

And during the creation of this music, I kept getting stronger and stronger, so I just kept writing and writing and writing, and a friend of mine gave me his apartment. He was a pianist who was here in New York. So he gave me his apartment in LA to write, and I stayed there for like 3 weeks. I didn't even hardly go home. And by the end of writing all of these—writing these songs, and I would write these massive diary—diary entries and actually had a—if—if I were a supernaturalist, I would have called it a transcended or supernatural experience. Not in the sense that I've experienced an entity.

In addition to helping Richard recover and reemerge into his life, the songwriting process resulted in the creation of his musical, which has been showcased throughout the United States. However, the music was more than that—it was Richard's refusal to die, to rebuild his spirit through his art, and his power to overcome adversity and not succumb to the realities and ravages of AIDS that brought him out of this period of pain and suffering and likely ensured his survival into middle age. I have purposely shared the story in its entirety because of its incredible power and because it perfectly exemplifies the will to survive evident among so many of the men of the AIDS Generation. In the end, for many there was simply a spirit to live and be defined by more than HIV.

This focus on living as demonstrated in this chapter, particularly in the story of Richard, is indicative of the positive attitudinal approaches enacted by so many men of the AIDS Generation. These approaches may help to explain why they are all long-term survivors. What is evident in so many of their life journeys is an underlying desire to live and face their disease head on. Julie Barroso (1996) describes this approach as focusing on living and indicates that this particular attitudinal approach, which incorporates having a positive attitude, planning for the future, and focusing on one's energies, helps to explain why these men have survived to this day. Kerry had a very interesting take on this idea and used the word "positive" as a means of building his will to live and survive and not as a way of being defeated. He used the words associated with his condition as part of his resilience:

I'm not a religious person but I'm spiritual. I always felt like there's, this is just housing something for me for now and there'll be another place to go.

And I think that's all helped me through. And I think it has a bigger part to play than people realize. I think one of the biggest things they did for us was to name it positive because it's positive, is a positive word. So as many times as I heard it, it was still a positive word. Do you know what I mean? Even though it was with relation to the disease, it's still positive. It's just the word has a connotation that's like "Come on, we can hang in there! We can—." So I'm willing to bet that there's a lot more than just we were young. I think we had some sort of happy, spiritual thing going on....And when I'm at my rock bottom, that phrase is what gets me through. When I just have to believe that and know it—and there've been plenty of times.

The Power of Escape

It would be short-sighted and misleading on my part only to demonstrate the proactive strategies that the men developed to cope with HIV. Also, after 20 years of research in the lives of gay men, I am abundantly aware of the role that sex, alcohol, and other drugs play in the lives of so many. I have followed patterns of risk associated with the confluence of substance use and sexual risk taking and recognize the synergistic risk associated with these behaviors (Halkitis et al., 2011). But I also recognize that for gay men, sexuality and sexual identity are central to how we define ourselves, and although substance use may not empower us to make the best decisions, it does provide a social lubricant for so many confronting the stigma and discrimination evident in our families, our communities, and our society at large.

In our previous volume *HIV + Sex*, based on the lives of HIV-positive gay and bisexual men collected via interviews in the late 1990s, David Purcell and his colleagues (2005) indicated that substance use serves several purposes in the sexual lives of HIV-positive men, including providing behavioral, cognitive, and emotional benefits. In this same volume, my colleagues and I (Halkitis & Wilton, 2005) indicate the multifaceted meaning of sex in the lives of HIV-positive men, including but not limited to an affirmation of self. This, then, is how I come to understand the role of sex and drugs in the lives of the men of the AIDS Generation. Although not all of the men partook in ongoing sexual adventurism or the use of substances, for some of the men of the AIDS Generation these behaviors were key to their lives as they ameliorated the ongoing reality of living with HIV (Halkitis, 2013). As a society, we look with a sense of compassion on those who create bucket lists. I ask the reader, then, to use the same orientation in considering the role of sex and substance use in the lives of the men of the AIDS Generation. Perhaps having sex with any men and feeling the numbing effects of substances were part their bucket lists. In the absence of any effective treatment, at a time of little hope, and surrounded by death, some of these men relied on sex and substances to manage their emotionally burdened lives.

Like his husband, Bobby, whose struggles with substances are described to follow, John turned to alcohol and drugs at even higher rates of use after his diagnosis. He concedes that his reliance on substances was, in part, to cope with being gay, and that in the presence of an HIV diagnosis, a death sentence in his perspective, there was even more impetus to use substances. Previous research has shown that the use of substances including alcohol functions to ameliorate the stigma associated with being gay (Parsons et al., 2004). When talking with John, these themes most clearly emerged in this section of our conversation:

PERRY: So as I'm listening to your story, I hear the use of the drugs and the alcohol to deal with the gay thing, right, now you've got the HIV thing, which compounds the gay thing, right? So why not?

JOHN: Yeah, why not?

PERRY: Why not?

JOHN: Oh, yeah, and why not, I was gonna die anyway?

PERRY: Right.

JOHN: So why not?

PERRY: You were gonna die in 2 years, 1 year, 3 years.

JOHN: Well, a year and a half is what that lady said.

PERRY: Right. Right.

JOHN: I knew what she meant. And within 6 months, Jeff [his partner at the time] said to me, "Ever since you found out you're a totally different person. You're out of control. You're an alcoholic; you're an addict. You either get the help you need or I'm leaving you." And I said, "Why should I? I'm gonna die anyway." And he left me. And I—then there was nothing holding me back then.

For the men of the AIDS Generation, the use of these substances is highly linked to sex. Sex, including unprotected sex, also provided an emotional connection, a validation of self, and an ability to perceive oneself as more than simply a vessel for HIV. Richard expressed it as follows:

But there was a certain acceptance I wanted through sex because I was positive. It was a reassurance that people still wanted to be with me. Do you know what I mean? So I think I did more sex after I was positive, I think

I was more sexual or tried to be more sexual because it was a way of people accepting me.

The reliance on sex and drugs did not always precede the HIV diagnosis. As is the case with Kerry, a longing for connection with others became more heightened in 1992, after it was determined that he was living with HIV:

> But there was a certain acceptance I wanted through sex because I was positive. It was a reassurance that people still wanted to be with me. Do you know what I mean? So I think I did more sex after I was positive; I think I was more sexual or tried to be more sexual because it was a way of people accepting me.

Of all of the men of the AIDS Generation, Andre's strategies for survival are most illustrative of reliance on sex and drugs as escape behaviors. For Andre, the voice of coping is primarily the voice of substance use. Andre, who first tested as part of his military training in 1986, began a career of alcohol and illicit drug use after his diagnosis that endured until 2001. This means of coping emerged immediately after his diagnosis, which coincided with graduation from military training:

> Uh, the night I was told was the first night I ever went and drank to get drunk. It was the night before graduation. Everyone celebrated because we were about to graduate. And I'd asked, "What will give me the most bang for my buck?" And someone said a triple shot of tequila. And we're on base. A drink—a shot was only $1.05. So for under $20.00 I got blotto. I blacked out. They had to wake me up the next morning for graduation. I grinned and made it through that. And from then until I went—after we went to the hospital—which took about a week—I was drunk pretty much all the time.

It is clear from Andre's story that this was the only means he had at his disposal for handling his diagnosis and what he feared what his imminent death: "Because like—because if I'm sober, if I'm not drunk—well, I've only got a couple more years left." These behaviors, for over a decade, led Andre, a gifted and talented man who had enormous potential in the military, to a life of public assistance, including living in shelters until shortly after 9/11 when he redirected the course of his life:

> I was in the shelter and, you know, the TV went out. The—what's going on? And finally, you know—the antenna was set up and they showed the

first tower falling. And we went outside. The shelter's in Long Island City, so we can see downtown Manhattan—and saw the second one fall. And it's like—no, the crash. Saw the first one fall. Yeah. And then people were volunteering to do cleanup over there and—at this point I'd made a deal. "If I get out of this shelter, I'll do something about my drinking."

After years of escape to numb the pain of his HIV status and the loss of four of his lovers, Gianni retold a similar story about 9/11: "I saw the towers fall and realized that I was still standing and needed to go on with my life, feel the pain, and become free to move on."

As is clearly delineated in his life history, the use of alcohol and casual sex preceded Bobby's diagnosis but was only heightened when he had to confront living with HIV:

> Um, so time passes, Bobby drinks, Bobby has one relationship with a genuinely really nice person but then Bobby also discovers the joys of having his own home computer and pornography delivered right into the confines of his home....I am smoking two packs cigarettes a day and drinking four nights a week.

This life of ongoing alcohol use persisted heavily until 1999, when he became extremely ill and went home to Louisiana to recover. Only after relapsing one more time did Bobby finally stop using alcohol: "Until Christmas Eve 2000 when I was arrested for my third DUI. Yeah, and committed, I didn't commit but I attempted to commit suicide, because I was so tired of the drinking and that was my last drink." This was more than a decade after seroconverting.

In the case of Tyronne, ongoing use of substances before, during, and after his diagnosis characterized his life, which he eventually addressed, after many years, in 2007. Like Bobby, Tyronne's understanding of his destructive behavior, which took the form of escape through substance use as well as selling his HIV medication to fuel his addiction, was tied to his childhood. Still, after a period of destructive behavior, Tyronne finally reexamined his life and undertook actions and behaviors to enhance his emotional well-being, which also had implications for his physical well-being.

These behavioral patterns of escape emerged somewhat differently for others who were less reliant on substances and sex prior to their own diagnoses and the AIDS crisis. For Ralph, drug use and associated sex emerged more after his move with Colin from Utah to San Francisco and after his diagnosis. The use of substances enabled Ralph to engage in the sexual scene of San Francisco but also to manage his emotions with regard to his partner's inevitable demise, which clearly made him confront his own mortality:

> Well, I had sex with all the people that died, I guess. Um, HIV people were having sex with HIV people, so um, uh, I mean, I didn't have a lot of sex because, again, I tell you, I didn't have much of a self-esteem so I wasn't very good at the art of picking up. I could pretend. When I was a bartender I was totally a character and that made things a lot easier because when you're a character you're acting a role, and I was good at that, but stepping away from that I was pretty bad. I did a lot of drugs. Drugs made things easier. Well, at the time too, Colin [his partner] was getting really sick and, um, I started doing a lot more drugs. I—you know, I remember he told me that and I went into rehab the next day.

These stories of sex and drugs demonstrate the struggles that many of the men of the AIDS Generation faced in trying to understand and manage their health conditions, as well as their sexual identities and places in the world. Monumental events in their lives, including worsening health conditions, witnessing ongoing deaths, the events of 9/11, and the aging process, functioned as catalysts to help each of these men achieve their sobriety. It would be simple and easy to judge their substance use and sexual behaviors and to label them as irresponsible, but as Bobby stated emphatically: "We weren't the only ones who did sex and drugs though." However, we were the ones with HIV circulating in our midst.

In light of a life-ending diagnosis, and in a world laden with homophobia and discrimination, the attempts of these men to escape and numb the pain are not only excusable but also understandable. Many of the men of my generation were simply trying to cope with the world around us, which was collapsing, literally and figuratively, as we all, too, were struggling to survive. In the end, as is evidenced in the following statement by John, making peace with all of these demanding realties in our lives was central to survival: "You know what, I'm gay, I'm—I'm living with AIDS, and I'm sober."

Conclusions

The men of the AIDS Generation developed and enacted many strategies to survive and be valuable, viable, and vibrant men to this day. All attended to their whole selves, including their physical well-being, emotional lives, and social engagement. In many, there was an undeniable desire to live—a spirit to survive. All of these ideas are captured beautifully in Hal's depiction of his holistic approach to surviving AIDS. To this point, he describes his actions and approaches postdiagnosis, in the midst and height of the crisis, as follows:

> I stopped drinking. I stopped having anal sex. I started eating right. I started exercising. I had a lot of safe sex with a lot of men. It was wonderful. People continued to die. The intimacy, the sexual intimacies that occurred in grief were so comforting. I saw shamans, I saw faith healers, as things progressed and I started getting sicker, I started really compound Q and riboflavin and all that stuff started coming out. And I was desperate to save my life so then people would say, "Oh, you're so courageous." And I'd be actually, I'm not. I'm terrified, but this is borne out of necessity. I don't want to die so I'm trying anything. And I was almost dead. I was planning my funeral. I was picking my music and that was at about 12 years in. And the drugs came out and I took the drugs, and within a month I was roller blading.

Asked why he was able to survive an HIV diagnosis in 1984, Hal simply said, "I've always been very Walt Disney about life. I've always believed that my knight in shining armor would show up on a horse and that I would live happily ever after." This reminds me of the words of Michael Callen (1990). When he was trying to make sense of his own survival in the first decade of AIDS, one of his explanations, in addition to luck and classic Coke, was the love a good man.

The men of the AIDS Generation confronted their disease but were not defined solely by their disease. Each one of the men described how his life evolved postdiagnosis. None defined the entirety of his identity solely by his disease. Those of us who have conducted work in the research or practice field occasionally meet HIV-positive individuals who use the expression "I am HIV." More often than not, such individuals lead their lives defined solely by their illness. The men of the AIDS Generation may be infected with HIV or they may have AIDS, but none indicated "I am HIV." Each man integrated his identity as a seropositive individual into the larger framework of his life and in turn undertook approaches to maintain his disease while proceeding forward with his life. None of the men stagnated.

The ideas reflected in this chapter also align with the seminal work of Julie Barroso (1996, 1997; Barroso et al., 1997). In her work, she proposes five dimensions for surviving AIDS: normalizing, focusing on living, taking care of oneself, being in relation to others, and triumphing. What is apparent in the stories of the men of the AIDS Generation is that each, in one way or another, manifested these dimensions. By attending to the physical, emotional, and social self and by building their sprit and facing HIV/AIDS "head on," these men enacted strategies that allowed them to survive.

I would also suggest that for some, their attempts at escape, via sex and substance use, were also a successful strategy that gave an additional dimension to their lives. Traditionally, reliance on sex and drugs is cast in a negative light and viewed as an avoidant coping strategy. I, however, view these behaviors as a release, an opportunity to escape the ongoing and demanding realties created by the AIDS epidemic at a time of little hope (Halkitis, 2013). Eventually, all of the men of the AIDS Generation were able to move beyond reliance on these strategies.

Moreover, all of these coping strategies helped the men of the AIDS Generation evolve into the men they are today. That is not to say that a life free from AIDS would not have been better. But some, like Gianni, reflected positively on his life and the strategies he had developed to over-come all of the struggles the AIDS epidemic inflicted. Relying again on popular music, as he often did in our conversation, Gianni said:

> Yeah, it was rough. It was horrible. It was awful. But it's like that Xtina [Christina Aguilera] song, "Fighter." "Makes me that much stronger, makes me that much wiser"—you know it made me learn how to fight for every-thing in my life. That's how I'm looking at it these days.

Finally, although the use of alcohol, other drugs, and sex as a means of coping is not traditionally viewed as an effective or active coping strat-egy, for the men of the AIDS Generation, these outlets provided a form of escape, a release, a decompression, from the ongoing onslaught of the AIDS epidemic. It is too simplistic to judge these behaviors as deviant or destructive unless you have walked in the shoes of these men.

In the end, there is probably no one set of strategies that explains the survival of each of the men of the AIDS Generation, as noted in the words of Ralph during the focus group:

> I wish I had a secret recipe to say why I feel like I've been successful with this disease. But I think it's luck and I think it's genetics. But I don't have a recipe that I could say do this and this will—I made wise choices. I exercise. I go to the doctor. I take my pills, but I don't think that's any recipe that

would work for everybody....People say, "Why is this happening? How come you're so successful?" You know? And I don't know what to say.

However, one thing is clear to me in dissecting these narratives. These men—the men of the AIDS Generation—had a will to survive, a drive, that brought them to my office for our meetings in 2012. Julie Barroso (1996) describes this dimension of survival as triumphing—coming to believe that AIDS was a blessing and that one could live with the disease. As we will see in the next chapter, living with AIDS has brought the men of the AIDS Generation into middle age.

CHAPTER 5 | And Then Middle Age
Gay Men Aging With HIV

I hope I'd be old before I died. That's what I always wanted—to get older. Like Robbie Williams—like that song says—you know, that British singer. Anyway that's what I wanted always. Now I'm 50.

THOSE ARE THE WORDS of Gianni when asked about getting older as a gay man, and more significantly as an HIV-positive gay man who is a long-term survivor. And so it is for the men of the AIDS Generation. In all likelihood and based on the current state of HIV treatments, many, if not all, of the men of the AIDS Generation will be old before they die, perhaps living a normal life expectancy, which is approximately age 79 for a 50-year-old man in the United States (Arias, 2011). The men of the AIDS Generation are entering "the autumn of their lives," as is the case for all those in middle age; however, for these men, this situation is a reversal of a cycle, because they have already lived through "the winter of their lives."

The age 50 marks a significant milestone in the lives of the men of the AIDS Generation. First, there is the cultural meaning assigned by our society to this golden year. It is, in fact, the year we can join the AARP (the American Association of Retired Persons, a powerful lobbying group in the United States). This age also marks a transitional period characterized by the onset of older adulthood and senescence of immune functioning, both of which hold powerful meaning for the men of the AIDS Generation, who have been managing and maintaining their physical, emotional, and social well-being for at least two decades.

The aging process is a complex phenomenon for all individuals, laden with physical, emotional, and social burdens (Gilmer & Aldwin, 2003). We all confront the physical manifestations, which intersect with our emotional and social well-being. However, becoming middle aged for the men of the AIDS Generation is an even more complicated matter because they have had a lifetime defined by more health complications and loss than that experienced by most other individuals. For HIV-positive gay men, 50 is both the new 40 and the new 60 (Halkitis, 2010b). This is due to the physical realities—the advances in treatment that have extended life—but also the chronic condition of HIV, which may accelerate the physical deterioration of the body, and the socio-emotional conditions brought forth by the possibilities of a future while they are also trying to reconcile and reconsider the actions, decisions, and missed opportunities of the past.

Entering middle age is indeed a mixed blessing for many of the men of the AIDS Generation. There is evidence both of happiness and awe and of struggle and confusion. For many of the men, there is obvious negotiation between the good and the bad, the joy and the pain, and ultimately the making of meaning. These are the elements that are further described in the chapter, summarized in part by Kerry's thoughts:

> I'm not complaining. I'm thrilled to be here. I have all my benefits paid for. I have a place. I have a 13-year-younger lover. All my lovers have been negative; they've all remained negative because of safe sex. So I don't want to sound like a downer at all. I just wish the gay community were a little bit more inclusive of us and had more respect for what we've been through. I feel like we're like the Vietnam vets.

As the men of the AIDS Generation emerge into middle age, they confront and must reconcile a life of painful and difficult memories. It is this struggle that is examined first in this chapter. In addition, what emerged in many of our conversations was the struggle some were facing to understand the process of aging, when this was outside their life expectations, and moreover how to make sense of this aging process. I consider this idea first and in relation to the concepts of legacy and survivor's guilt, and with regard to the emotions associated with aging. The men also described and considered the physical manifestations and experiences associated with the aging process both in relation to and separate from their HIV status; these experiences were very real and tangible and also are considered in this chapter. Finally, and most clearly, the men of the AIDS Generation voiced their thoughts with regard to being older gay men in a youth-obsessed society, as well as their struggle in understanding the perpetuation of the epidemic in a new generation of young gay men. An exploration of these ideas concludes the chapter. These myriad conditions, some life affirming and future oriented and others fraught with fear and ambivalence, are evidenced among many aging HIV-positive gay men who are long-term survivors, including those beyond the borders of the United States, as recently noted in the work conducted by Owen and Catalan (2012) with gay men in London.

Throughout this volume I have referred to the men of the AIDS Generation as long-term survivors. They each have managed to maintain their lives into middle age and after at least two decades of living with HIV. But like all humans, their lives will not exist in perpetuity; they too will cease to exist at some point, a matter that reemerges as the men begin to age. This understanding is critical as we examine the experiences of the men of the AIDS Generation. To this point, I am reminded of an essay written by Mark Doty (1995), who, reflecting on the loss of his partner to AIDS, suggested (p. 11), "The world has one long term survivor, which is the world." This statement must be held closely as we examine the aging process of the men of the AIDS Generation.

A Life of Painful Memories

For many of these men, like Jackson, whose identity is in part defined by his involvement in AIDS activism, the process of aging ignites, fuels, and strengthens memories of what has transpired over the last three decades of their lives, the memories of those loved and lost to a health crisis that has taken the lives of hundreds of thousands of gay men:

> And they were all so vivid and so terrible that I realized my life is going to be a struggle between, you know, honoring the fallen soldiers and the memory of the time and ACT UP and what I'm holding in my heart and trying to find some measure of peace within myself so that I can walk away—you know, live my life. You know, and that—but that's just going to be life.

Patrick too expressed similar thoughts when the men of the AIDS Generation met as a group in September 2012, as he was reminded of what had transpired in his own life:

> But, um, I'll tell you what brings it back. And I do think about the—I don't think it happens sometimes until a month ago when they had the AIDS conference in Washington, DC, and I saw pictures of the quilt. It was like seeing the Towers on fire again. [Hal: Yup.] It brought it—when I saw the pictures of the quilt, I was like ahhhh! It was sickening. [Eddie: Yeah.] I mean the hair stood up on the back of my neck and I thought it did happen and I did know these people. And it all came back. And I remembered that quilt thing.

Even if they did not directly experience this abundance of loss to this gay men's health crisis in the 1980s and 1990s, all of the men were no more than one person removed from the circumstances. In the case of Bobby, these experiences were not drawn from his own life while he was a young man coming of age in Tennessee and Louisiana, but from that of his husband, John, who emerged as an adult in New York City. When the men gathered for the focus group meeting, Bobby described it as follows:

> But anyway, John, my husband, will describe exactly what you just said and he will respond in exactly the same way. There was our wedding day and he said, "I wish I could find that black book and so I could at least name these people. You know, say their names out loud because they're not gonna be here." And he said we're talking scores of people. He was in advertising in Manhattan in the '80s. I mean, you figure it out. So I had the luxury, I guess is the word, of not being here. So I—I didn't.... .

Experiencing these memories is part of the normal life cycle and emerges for most individuals as they enter the later stages of life. However, for the men of the AIDS Generation, memories fraught with loss and despair may be even more vivid and challenging to negotiate, and the healthy negotiation of these psychosocial struggles is key as these men understand their past and their legacies.

An Eriksonian Framing of the Aging Process

During middle age, according to developmental psychologist Erik Erikson (1980), individuals confront the life struggle of generativity versus stagnation. In this period, most individuals take stock of their places in the world and what they have accomplished that benefits other people. Individuals consider and examine what they have provided to their homes and their communities, and a healthy resolution of this conflict will allow one to successfully navigate into the later stage of life and perhaps resolve that ensuing conflict with integrity rather than despair. Later, I also will come to understand this idea as a struggle with legacy.

In addition, as noted by Erikson, Erikson, and Kivinick (1986), this period of life is marked by a reexamination of the earlier stages; in a sense individuals reexamine and rework the life of the past while navigating through the life of the present. In effect, during the middle age life cycle the men of the AIDS Generation were immersed in at the time of our interviews, the tension they were experiencing between the syntonic and dystonic forces (i.e., generativity versus stagnation) was also being complemented by a reexamination of the life stages of the past.

The notion of this Eriksonian tension is one that has resonance in framing the memories of the men with whom I spoke. For Bobby, an educator familiar with this psychological theory, an Eriksonian perspective is how he contextualizes his own life of memories and aspirations:

As a young boy, I was very precocious. Very. Off-the-charts smart in reading and math, with an amazing memory for all sorts of facts. So I grew up with this idea that I was/am somehow destined for greatness. As I grew older, turns out I wasn't such a freakin' genius after all. I'm a fairly smart guy, I suppose, but nothing on the scale of that early promise. This has led to more than a small amount of disappointment, felt by myself and by others. So I continue in the process of shedding those early unrealistic expectations and deciding what I want to be remembered for most. My childhood created wild daydreams of the presidency, multiple Academy Awards, reaching at least the third round at Wimbledon. My adulthood is creating reasonable and no less admirable daydreams of a legacy based more realistically on matters directly in my control: my relationships with family and friends, my passion for my career, and the example John and I can set in our marriage. This puts me squarely in Erickson's "integrity versus despair" conflict. When I remember who I really am, what gifts I was given that I can use, I explore and celebrate my own integrity. When I regress to dwelling on the fictional me, who was going to graduate from medical school at 19, that's a foolproof recipe for despair.

It is clear from Bobby's statement that his current struggle to understand his own place in the world—the tension of middle age—was being realized, in part through a reassessment of the previous period of his life.

Unfortunately, as helpful as Erikson's model may be in framing the conflicts of middle age, the theory is laden with the biases of its time, including the heteronormative nature of the paradigm. The theory relies heavily on heterosexual partnering and emphasizes procreation and childrearing, which until recently have not been a circumstance common to many gay men. Thus, using a very traditional interpretation of this framework, one could envision more pronounced struggles for gay men as they enter middle age. I choose to view it more broadly, and despite its shortcoming, the theory nonetheless speaks to the sensibility of all adults as they enter middle age—that of making sense of one's contributions to the world.

For the men of the AIDS Generation, the conflicts of middle age may have less to do with reproduction and more to do with a life unraveled because of the AIDS epidemic. As we have seen in the previous chapters, for each one of the men with whom I spoke, the earlier stage of psychosocial development—that of young adulthood—was interrupted by a health crisis that thrust these men emotionally forward into the last stage of life as they were confronting their life-threatening illness. At a time when these young men should have been negotiating their places in the world, they instead were confronted with the possibility of dying by age 30 or 35 or 40. However, they did not die and now find themselves at or around age 50 trying to make sense of their contributions to the world as middle-aged HIV-positive men. I believe that despite the harrowing circumstances, the men of the AIDS Generation have managed these life struggles with finesse and that the manner in which they have handled their life circumstances informs a mode of resilience, which I will fully address in the final chapter.

This is all to say that it is quite appropriate, at this developmental stage, for men of the AIDS Generation, in fact all men of this age group, to actively engage with their memories of their life experiences. It is through this process that they begin to negotiate and understand how they have made their life choices and what they have contributed to the world. In fact, this process is posited to be easier at this stage of life than in earlier periods, and a body of research has shown that older adults show more emotionally gratifying memory distortion for past choices than younger adults (Kennedy, Mather, & Carstensen, 2004; Mather & Johnson, 2000), in effect easing the impact of reliving life experiences. Said differently, our life choices may appear better (perhaps less problematic) in the context of middle age. Even the harrowing memories of loss, which were expressed by so many of the men with whom I spoke, were contextualized within a larger framework of legacy and understanding of one's own life.

It's About Legacy.. .

The rekindling of memories and understanding of the past may also be understood within another framework, that of an "existential crisis of legacy." The extant literature on the concept of legacy is one that is beginning to emerge, especially as it relates to those with life-threatening illnesses. The work of Claudia Sadler-Gerhardt and J. Grant Hollenbach (2011) provides a robust clear perspective for understanding the issue of legacy confronted by the men of the AIDS Generation. To this point, they state (p. 1):

> Legacy is popularly understood in today's culture as referring to the idea of leaving something of oneself behind for future generations. Frequently legacy has been understood in two primary ways. First, it can indicate a material legacy—that appropriation of material and familial possessions to family or friends after one's death, or a financial bequest to an institution or cause. Second there is the biological legacy—that inheritance of genetic traits with susceptibility to certain health conditions passed through the generations. However, the phenomenon of legacy as an aspect of aging or terminal illness has been understudied in the end of life literature, especially from the perspective of transmitting values and beliefs to loved ones left behind.... .

The last sentence of this statement is the one that speaks mostly clearly to the men of the AIDS Generation. As noted by Doka (2009), as people age they struggle with whether others will remember them and grapple with whether their lives had meaning. In the face of impending death, they search for a meaning and their places in the world (Moremen, 2005), a condition that has been proposed to be more pronounced for those with life-threatening diseases (Chochinov et al., 2005). And the fear of death may be informed by one's concern that one's life has been meaningless (Rayburn, 2008). For the men of the AIDS Generation, there had been an extended period of a death expectation at a very young age. Thus, while death was looming, as it does naturally for older adults, there had not been a life trajectory or an abundance of years of living to inform each of their legacies. Imagine a 25-year-old who is not confronted with HIV and his impending death. To what extent does this young man attend to his life accomplishments and legacy? He likely does not attend to such matters and has a normal life process at that point in his life. For the men of the AIDS Generation, however, there was an abnormal and unnatural life process. These men were forced to confront their legacies at an unnatural time—at a time when they should have been focused on beginning their life paths that would eventually and naturally bring them to a point decades later when they could, as nature plans, confront the issue of legacy. The men with whom I spoke and thousands like them did not experience this rite of passage.

At the same time, when confronted with facing the possibility of their impending death, many of these men undertook actions that helped to affirm and establish their legacies, although I doubt this was a conscious effort at the time—rather, these were actions that informed their survival. Still, to this point, many did, at an early age, undertake actions that in middle age clearly speak to their legacies. Hal was adamant and steadfast in the belief about his legacy based on his life course: "I've personally raised hundreds of thousands for various AIDS organizations. I am a pioneer in AIDS education. I have met every goal I have set." For Richard, who faced death more closely than any of the other men with whom I spoke, efforts at that time were directed toward his AIDS blog and his music, which at the time helped him cope with his disease, but which, at this point in his life, also inform his legacy. He describes it as follows:

> I addressed it when I wrote the song "Save Me a Seat," which is about my own memorial service—which became the opening number.... In the lyric, I say, after the service is over:
> "Then I'll get to do something you cannot do
> I'll follow you home, every one of you
> Then on a day when you feel lost or hurt
> Go to the kitchen and get some dessert
> Then sit at the table and eat
> Just remember to save me a seat."
> I suppose it has something to do with legacy, but it's more a yearning to not be forgotten. A fear that I'll have done so little in life that it will be as if I never existed

As noted in Richard's words, a yearning not to be forgotten speaks to his legacy. His legacy is the transmission of the ideas, values, and beliefs that he shared through his writing and his art that will exist to inform our social condition for many years after the epidemic is resolved. This too is how Christopher understands his legacy and, more to the point, his struggle with legacy. When asked to comment on the idea of legacy, Christopher said:

> That's a really tough question, at least for me. Half the time I never know what I want to do in the next 5 minutes, let alone what kind of legacy I want to leave. Two of my friends that both passed away from HIV/AIDS had a following poem printed on their prayer cards or in their memorial service programs. I often get it out and read it and I keep doing what I can to do—those things. Some days are harder than others. In my life, I've struggled with a lot of self-worth issues, sexual compulsion/addiction and depression, among other challenges. I try to make an effort every day to improve myself and be a better husband, a better son—son-in-law, a better brother—brother in-law, a better uncle, a better boss, a better friend, and overall a better example of a human being.

Here also, we can see the workings of Eriksonian theory as Christopher considers his generativity—the type of man he will be remembered as—and frames it within the context of previous life events, actions, and experiences (i.e., his past compulsions and addictions). In addition, although Hunter and Rowles (2005) would suggest that such transmission, as noted in the words of Richard and Christopher, is to loved ones left behind, I would suggest a broader conception that legacy involves a transmission of values and beliefs to individuals but also society at large. Interestingly, in the case of Richard, legacy is primarily understood through his music, and such an approach to legacy does hold historical roots in the field of music therapy (West, 1994). Recall that at the time, this expression, this music, was the therapy that sustained Richard. Now it is also part of his legacy.

It is in this voice that John also came to understand his legacy—that of the perpetuation of his behavior and values—which can also be framed as his negotiation between the tension of generativity and despair. John, who had recently married Bobby at the time of our second meeting, described his wedding vows, which reflect his legacy as his survival and also of the values that he and Bobby transmit to their loved ones:

> I see in you a man like myself who realized that no matter how bad things got, there was always someone worse off who could use our help and benefit from our experience; you even made a career out of it. I hope to be remembered as a man who turned his biggest obstacles into his greatest assets

and was able to proudly share them as well as his experience, strengths, hopes, and most of all his love with his family, friends, and community.

The men of the AIDS Generation established their legacies, unconsciously, during their formative years, when first confronted with AIDS, and throughout their lives through the dignity they demonstrated in combating AIDS. Their legacies are not indicated by awards, wealth, or accumulated objects but rather by their strategies for survival. As young men fighting a deadly virus, they undertook actions to help them cope with the illness. Establishing a legacy was hardly what they had in mind at the time—survival was the goal. This too was the case for my partner Robert, who refocused his journalistic efforts on learning and writing about HIV as a means of survival for himself and his community and these days is remembered as a pioneer in AIDS journalism. The act of survival as legacy is also evidenced in the world of Antoine, who now transmits these values to a new generation of gay men living with the virus. When asked about his life and what he has accomplished, Antoine reflected as follows:

> I mean, I appreciate you doing the work that you're doing because as you know, 30 years ago, none of these books would have been published—or been mainstream. And you could not have the slate and an office of this—I was looking out this window, and I watched the evolution of this park because I can remember 18, 19, sitting out there coming from Paradise Garage, sitting out there deciding are we going to go to Reese Beach or are we going to go home? Or go to Fire Island or wherever, you know. So—and it's also to those that are coming up—because even as I said to a young man who was, 3 years ago, who was 19 and was positive, and when I told him that I was and how long I was positive, how long I've been positive, I said to him, "I want you to go back and get your GED. And after you get that GED, I want you to go to college because your life is not over."

Like all of the men of the AIDS Generation, Antoine has been surviving HIV his entire adult life. In fact, Antoine comes to understand the lifelong struggle to survive as his legacy when he describes the idea as follows: "This is the only thing in my life that I've had longer than anything else. Other than a relationship with my family." So, too, the previous excerpt demonstrates how in his attempt to negotiate this current Eriksonian life struggle, Antoine is drawing on his prior life stages and using that point of reexamination as a means of guiding a new generation of young gay men.

As the men of the AIDS Generation survive this epidemic and enter middle age, issues of legacy become more pronounced. This is due in part to the fact that many of the men did not expect to be middle aged. So after a lifetime seeking to survive this epidemic, the men arrive at middle age and begin to understand this issue for what it actually is and represents, and moreover grapple with how to establish and understand their legacies.

This awareness of legacy during middle age is quite different from the unconscious understanding the men had of it at younger ages. In this regard, I am reminded of a very dear colleague, an HIV-positive man is his 50s who has been living with the virus most of his adult life, and who on more than one occasion asked me if I believed that our work in the field of HIV prevention would be remembered in history books. His question, which always elicited in me a sense of great sorrow, is a manifestation of his own struggle with legacy. In contrast to my colleague, John seems to understand his legacy, and so do those who love him. John retold the story of his nephew, his namesake, who described his uncle and his uncle's legacy as follows:

> He started by saying his name and that he had the rare privilege of "shadowing" me for the last 19 years and then he went on to describe what that was like. He described a proud, gay, sober alcoholic living with HIV—an uncle who took him as a young teenager to a Long Island middle school to hear him speak about his life living with HIV, growing up gay and overcoming alcoholism and addiction, an uncle whose volunteer work as an EMT inspired him to join the Southampton Volunteer Ambulance. By the time he was done, I was in tears.... I think I covered what I'd like my legacy to be.

These words can also be understood in relation to John's tension between generativity and despair, which, in his case, appears to be resolving in an effective manner.

In the end, what I learned in talking with the men of the AIDS Generation is that their stories of survival are in fact their legacies. As noted by Elizabeth Hunter (2007, p. 313) in her work with women, "...legacy emerges as a means of passing on the essence of one's life, in particular one's values and beliefs." For the men of the AIDS Generation, their commitment to living, as well as all of the actions they undertook to survive, is their legacy. In these actions they demonstrated their values—importance of life and how we each must embrace every moment we are given. These values and actions, which they have transmitted to their own social circles and to the world in turn, establish their legacies, because this strength and courage defines them. These life-affirming experiences and their will to live, which also permeated the earlier stages of their lives, appear front and center as many of the men experience the syntonic and dystonic forces that accompany middle age. To this point, Patrick said:

> I have been thinking about this quite a bit in the last few years. When I talk to close friends and family, their feedback is clearly that my biggest accomplishments have been my survival, strength, and ability to live successfully in this city.

Their contributions to the world are remarkable insomuch as we can learn from their life experiences and how each of these men, and many others like them, managed a life-threatening condition while maintaining his integrity and viability. What we learn from these stories of survival in the midst of despair and little hope informs a model of resilience, which will be explored in the final chapter of this book. For Detroit-born Eddie, sharing his story served this purpose but also served as inspiration to himself after years of negotiating substance use, an affirmation of his life as on older gay HIV-positive man, and a testament to his legacy:

> One of the ways I think that I sort of am able to be happy about getting older and sort of feel great about myself is by doing things like this. I think really in my opinion all we really have is our stories. And for the fact that you can put a book like this together and sort of celebrate all of our unique stories is just like—is a way for me to sort of continue to—to feed off of that sort of energy. And it just continues to amaze me just being in this room today and hearing all your stories and talking about this; it continues to energize me.

When I was first conceiving this volume, it was this idea of legacy that I held in the front of my mind. Besides simply documenting this critical aspect of my history, and of our history, I hoped to glean from these stories insights that can benefit anyone confronting a challenging health condition. I believe deeply and I have come to know that the men of the AIDS Generation, who came of age in the 1970s and 1980s, and who have survived the epidemic, are role models. The stories of these men and their strategies for combating the physical, emotional, and social challenges of the epidemic provide a gateway for understanding how individuals managed their lives in the era of AIDS, and provide a health context by which to explore and understand how individuals cope with chronic and life-threatening diseases. Similar thinking was shared by Richard:

> I also think all of us Lazarus people have a very important life story and message that is important to our culture and to our society. We've been through—it's like going through a war and surviving a war. And having experiences that are valuable, a certain kind of wisdom that comes from being a Lazarus person.

The value placed on the lives of these men and those who they inspire also informs their legacy. I am not alone in my firm conviction that these are the bravest, most beautiful men of their time. Others in their lives, others who know where our values should reside, share my beliefs. Bobby indicated this idea when he said:

> And there are people who will e-mail you or call you and say, "I just wanted to let you know how much I respect you." How much I—what did I do? A little bit of HIV 24 years and you beat cancer and this is a big deal to people. We're kind of going to the bank and doing our daily routine. We're nobody special but people invest us with some kind of energy or some kind of power.

Even for Kerry, who struggles to negotiate the meaning of his life, participating in these discussions did help him realize his contributions to the world: "I don't feel recognized. Like this makes me feel recognized, acknowledged. I feel like my life wasn't for nothing. Do you know what I mean?"

As I enter middle age, this struggle with my own legacy has been front and center for close to 2 years. I have come to understand this particular work, this book, as more than another facet of my research program, but rather as my own personal legacy as well as the legacy of the men of the AIDS Generation. I think, too, that my colleague David France and the leaders of the ACT UP group in New York and the Treatment Action Group (TAG) were directed by similar internal motivations in the making of *How to Survive a Plague*. This is our history, our legacy, our story—it needs to be told and, more importantly, we need to understand it. We chose to tell our stories, which is the most common way aging individuals understand their lives and their legacies (Hunter, 2007; McAdams, 1993).

...But Not About Survivor's Guilt

One understanding became very clear to me as I was talking with the men of the AIDS Generation in our one-on-one meetings, in our focus groups, and in my interactions with them throughout the course of writing this volume. The voice of guilt is not a voice that emerged in their understanding of their lives. In late October 2012, I engaged with the men of the AIDS Generation over e-mail to help clarify my thinking about this matter, and the passages shared in this section are drawn from those interactions.

Early in the epidemic, the idea of survivor's guilt surfaced in the HIV counseling and behavioral literature. This construct was featured in Walt Odets' *In the Shadow of the Epidemic* (1995). In this work, Odets examines the guilt of HIV-negative men, men of my generation, who somehow managed to avoid infection with the virus and, because of what they had witnessed in their communities and social circles, had developed a sense of guilt around their serostatus. To this point, Odets posits a psychological epidemic among gay men based on observation in his own practice. In 1995 (p. 20) he wrote, "I have seen innumerable examples of psychological problems among gay men that seven years ago would have been unusual and noteworthy, that are now so common that they almost pass without comment." For HIV-negative gay men, Odets attributes this state to self-silencing—feelings of disenfranchisement from the gay community and isolation from HIV-positive men (p. 21).

I asked the men of the AIDS Generation about this construct as I was writing this section of the book, and Ryan, who for a period of time worked at GMHC, said:

> As for neg men's survivor's guilt, I honestly have no patience for that. These are men who never went to the war, and therefore, can't have "survivor's guilt" in my opinion. They may feel loss and sadness in their lives as a result of losing so many around them, but I don't believe this is really guilt.

I agree with Ryan. The concept of survivor's guilt is not one that I have readily accepted, and it has limited support in the empirical literature. The construct is similar, in my view, to "bug chasing" (i.e., intentionally seeking to become infected with HIV) that has garnered much more attention than merited. It is a sensational and somewhat sexy construct, one that therapists and clinicians have discussed in the literature (e.g., Gabriel, 1994; Koetting, 1996; Valente, 2003), but also one that has more limited support in the scientific literature as an actual phenomenon and construct. The construct has also permeated at least one artistic response—in Jonathan Larson's *Rent*, the character Mark Cohen, who is uninfected, relies on his work as a documentarian and filmmaker to cope with the "guilt" of his well-being while his friends, Angel, Mimi, Roger, and Tom Collins, are living with HIV.

In Odets' view (1995, p. 21), the concept of survivors' guilt is one that also has applicability and manifests among HIV-positive men who are long-term survivors, men like those you have come to know in these pages. In 1999 (p. 35), Jose Catalan also wrote, "Finally a new version of survivor's guilt can arise in the wake of new combination therapies; if only those who perished had access to these new treatments!" Perhaps this is an even more challenging and misplaced understanding of survivor's guilt. I asked the men of the AIDS Generation cohort to comment on this idea. When Ralph was asked if this was a condition he experienced or experiences, he refuted the idea and instead said:

> Survivor pride—my strength and ability to survive keep me going. Anyone who died I'm sure would want me to as long as I can. Guilt? For living? Nope!

Similarly, Richard added, "I was just happy to survive. I'm not much of a guilt person, anyway," to which Hal added, "I agree. I don't feel guilty. Just perplexed sometimes." I think the statements of these three men are key to understanding the social and emotional states of the men of the AIDS Generation as they age. Yes, they are in awe of living; yes, they are at a crossroads as they embark on middle age; yes, they lived through a life where an early death was expected; and yes, they have witnessed loss and devastation. But these conditions are not ones that evoke feelings of guilt. These are not negative conditions; they are life statements that align more with a struggle to understand their legacies—their places in the world—as has been previously noted. Patrick, a dancer who is now a personal trainer, was very animated in his response in this regard:

> Ha! Survivor's guilt. As if I don't have enough on my plate already I should think I have guilt about being healthy again? I miss my friends dearly but I know I survived because I have many things to teach and learn. A Course in Miracles clued me in early on that guilt is useless and a physically and mentally draining emotion.... I have no time for guilt. Except maybe when I eat the last piece of cheesecake.

Ryan also was very articulate in his response about survivor's guilt, in which he demonstrates the ideas that I have proposed:

> I personally don't believe in survivor's guilt for poz men. I think it is something else, but not guilt. It is gratitude; it is remorse and loss for those who died; it is a sense of how it could have just as easily been us who didn't make it to today, had it not been our very lucky timing and the treatments that became available. I don't believe this is guilt. We came back from the war and have the trauma associated with that war.

Even for Bobby, who did not witness the loss and devastation noted by the other men as he was coming of age in the South, outside the AIDS epicenter in New York City, the idea of survivor's guilt did not resonate with his understanding of his life path:

> I am not personally familiar with the concept of survivor guilt. It's never crossed my mind to wonder why I lived and so many others didn't. I know that for many years after testing HIV positive, my choices were not the choices of a man who wanted to live. So I survived my self-destructive behaviors, while others who went the macrobiotic/yoga/holistic/etc. route died. That means to me that I am less in control of my destiny than I'd like to believe. I don't surrender my agency because of this, but I balance the efficacy of my own actions with the chances and choices that the universe has in store for me. I got good genes, a set of emotional/personality traits that somehow lets me not worry too much and a bunch of good luck.

Jackson was particularly insightful in reframing the ideas regarding survivor's guilt, which he outright rejects:

> I wonder sometimes "why fortune smiles on some and lets the rest go free" [a lyric from the Eagles song "The Sad Cafe"], but I wouldn't describe it as survivor's guilt. I also reject the notion of HIV survivor's guilt, because surviving tragic events like a war or a mass shooting have identifiable, finite endpoints. Being an HIV survivor is less definable and may not even be accurate.

Instead, like Bobby, he wonders why he has survived this epidemic, which he refers to as an HIV survivor's curiosity:

> I do have "survivor's deep curiosity." Like Bobby, and some of the others who have responded, I think I'm fortunate to have good genes, a

personality that allows me to face difficulties and crises in a healthy way, family support, insurance, great doctors, etc., but it may be I was infected with a weak strain of the virus or happen to have a physiological makeup that is able to deal with the virus, which some would call "just dumb luck." I do a lot of work to stay healthy with a clear knowledge that there were people who worked a hell of a lot harder than I did who didn't survive.

In the end, if Jackson experiences any guilt, it is not about his own survival, drawing from his experience watching *How to Survive a Plague*:

> Peter Staley, in the amazing documentary of AIDS activism *How to Survive a Plague*, raises a question about walking away from the war. It stayed with me. If I feel any guilt, it wouldn't be about surviving with HIV, but I often ask myself why I'm not the same fierce, in-your-face, committed activist I once was.

Finally, I turn to John's story. John experienced his reaction to the many losses, including that of his first husband, to AIDS as a type of guilt. However, he, like the others, does not engage with this conception any longer. Once John confronted his substance use, he realized that his life was a blessing, and that guilt was what he was experiencing:

> The death sentence I thought I was given turned this functioning alcoholic into an out-of-control alcoholic/addict and I spent countless hours alternating between wondering when my turn would come and feeling guilty that I was still alive while other HIV-poz men who were leading healthier lives were dying. Once I got sober in 1992, my attitude changed considerably mainly because I got off the pity pot and developed an attitude of gratitude....I lost six of my closest gay male friends to AIDS, men who were role models, confidants, my "gay" family, men who I expected to share my life with along with many of the hundreds of friends who died from this disease, so yes, I still wonder why I am still here and they are gone, but I no longer feel the guilt that I used to feel. I just feel very, very blessed.

Yet even though the men of the AIDS Generation did not wholeheartedly embrace the idea of survivor's guilt, they did accept the notion that some others could have feelings that could be construed as guilt, and that these emotions should not be judged. To this point, Christopher commented as follows, indicating that survivor's guilt may not be driven by emotional states but rather by social programming:

> I don't think the act of surviving is wrong, nor is it a crime someone should feel guilty for, but I'm suggesting people often do feel guilty anyway even when they've done nothing wrong.

Also, Richard noted that we should not judge, even if he does not experience guilt:

> I do believe those who experience guilt, straight or gay—mostly because feelings are not right or wrong. They just are. And also, feelings aren't fact. So, a cry from the heart helps clear the air.

This discourse on survivor's guilt makes it clear that this is a concept these men do not wholeheartedly embrace as they emerge into middle age. Rather, their thoughts reflect how they understand their places in the world and why they actually have survived the epidemic. This is not to say that some older gay men, positive or negative, may not experience this emotional state; perhaps instead the preponderance of this construct in our collective narrative is driven by the beliefs of a subset of empowered and visible voices, rather than the reality of the many.

In hearing these ideas regarding survivor's guilt, I am reminded of my own journey over the last 30 years. I think often of Jim, Tony, Robert, Rick, and Cameron. I think of their deaths. I think of my life and how much richer it is having known these men. I feel the pain of their deaths. But never do I feel guilty to be a healthy middle-aged man. I am grateful and I live to honor their memories, not to retreat into isolation because of some misplaced selfish sense of guilt.

The Social and Emotional Rollercoaster of Aging

As these men of the AIDS Generation enter middle age, the complexities of life abound. Each of the men of the AIDS Generation with whom I spoke expressed an overwhelming sense of awe and wonder that they were entering or had entered middle age. To this point, Eddie indicated: "And I think the testament to this is that we're all still here. And we all, regardless of whatever we've been through, seems like we're all still happy to be alive." The fact is that each and every one of them embraced the spirit to live and survive even in the darkest moments of AIDS and prior to 1996, before any true and effective treatment became available. Richard described it as follows:

> And I labeled this part of my life "living in the bonus round." The ding! The bell went off; life was over. And now time speeds up, prizes are better, and you have to keep going until they ding the bell again.

The process of making sense of one's life is a complicated and emotional undertaking for these men—a task that required introspection and the rekindling of memories. And for some, like John, this is an active process in which he obtained mental health support to relive the memories, process the experiences, and ultimately move forward with his life. As noted earlier, this process of memory making allows the men to understand their lives and their legacies.

> And still it is the hardest thing and also psychologically, I've been seeing a psychiatrist once every 3 months and it's just a check-up on me. And he's been trying to get me to remember that the choices I've made all connect back to that bump in the road because I've done such a fantastic job of forgetting about it. But I have to remember that every choice that I've made since then has led me to where I am. And so when I get to a very stressed-out or depressed place or fearful place, I have to backtrack and think, "What is this coming from?" I know it's coming back from the AIDS. I know it's— and once I kind of figure it out for myself whatever it is and maybe have a drink or something, then it's okay.

Making sense of getting older is a process in which all of the men with whom I spoke are actively engaged. It is occurring and evolving for all of them as I write this volume. In most other matters that I discussed with the men, there was generally a consistent voice that emerged—a set of ideas and themes that permeated almost all of the conversations, such as the "myth of two" or experiences of death for the last 30 years. This is because the men with whom I spoke had years to process these life experiences, to understand them, to contextualize them, and in effect to recall their thoughts, feelings, and actions. And in this regard, a collective voice emerged for many of the topics. However, the process of aging and making sense of what it means to be an older man is the one area that was less well formed, perhaps more poorly understood because it is ongoing, and thus what emerged from the conversations was not one set of clear collective voices, but rather a smattering of ideas that were still being processed and developed. Making sense of getting older included a recognition of the value of life, of the possibility of a normal life expectancy, and of hope, but also of frustration and of the angst associated with a new set of deaths—deaths not associated with AIDS but with the normal life process and aging. It is a time laden with a new set of social and emotional conditions with which the men of the AIDS Generation must grapple.

Owen and Catalan (2012) report similar findings. Some of the 10 older HIV-positive gay men they interviewed regarded aging as an opportunity to continue to achieve life goals, whereas others expressed greater ambivalence. The researchers posit that these differences emerged due to the history each man possessed with regard to the disease—in other words, his life course in relation to HIV. In this regard, Rosenfeld, Bartlam, and Smith (2012) also suggest that if we are truly to fully understand how HIV has affected the generation of gay boomers, men of the AIDS Generation, adapting a life course perspective is critical. In their view (p. 257), if we are truly to capture both the resilience and despair experienced by these men, we must expand our understanding of "...how later life is shaped by the intersection between historical events, personal biography, and social and community ties." For adults who have lived with HIV for extended periods and have experienced the cycles of hope and despair, the process of aging may be affected by a sense of psychological depletion (Schonnesson, 2002). Moreover, as has been the case throughout their lives, the men of the AIDS Generation, like all those living with HIV, live with a certain level of uncertainty, including but not limited to the long-term effects of treatment, the extent to which one's immune system is fully restored, and how to understand "chronic" in the new framing of HIV as a chronic disease (Siegel & Lekas, 2002). All of these conditions perpetuate a state of ongoing anxiety in the lives of these men, and thus making sense of one's life as one ages cannot be separated from these ongoing emotional and physical conditions that shape the lives of the men of the AIDS Generation.

In this section we examine how the men of the AIDS Generation understand and express what it means to be an older man and how to make sense of it. One need only consider the words of Hal to understand why this process—this meaning making around aging—is so challenging:

It was because I just—I don't know if it's a habit but I always assume I'm gonna predecease my family and because of having angioplasty 11 days ago and lipid issues and blood pressure issues I often will think I'm gonna predecease my siblings and my partner and I may make it to 65; that seems on a reasonable number based on the information we have now scientifically. But then I also look at the fact that for 28 years I've been in and out of hospitals and sick and dying and I don't.

Reevaluation

As shown in Gianni's words, which opened this chapter, and in my discussion about the spirit in Chapter 4, for many of the men of the AIDS Generation, there was always a hope that a life as an older adult would emerge. However, as shown here in the voice of Richard, confronting a life-threatening condition required a realignment of values and beliefs:

> I was diagnosed 20 years ago [begins to sound more emotional, tearful] and I refer—the one thing I think that we all have in common that we have talking about something positive is that we all kind of seen that edge of death, faced death and walked through it and then come out the other side. It changed my perspective on life when I thought I was gonna die. When I thought I was on my deathbed the things that I thought were important suddenly I realized were not important. And the very few things that really were important start to magnify themselves: friends, people that I love around me, taking care of others. And, uh, sometimes the battle is just so tough, I just get tired, of fighting. And it feels like an extravagant effort to stay alive sometimes.

For Richard and for many of the men of the AIDS Generation, being forced to confront death required a realignment of values and is part of their identities as they enter the later stages of life. Perhaps it is one of the most beneficial byproducts of this epidemic for my generation of gay men, whether we are HIV-positive or HIV-negative. We learned to appreciate life and not get muddled in the web of irrelevancies. In Project Gold, a 59-year-old who had been living with HIV since 1985, expressed it as follows: "I wouldn't be who I am without all of this. It's given me character and also much more understanding about how to make decisions."

This condition of reassessment is not unique to the men of the AIDS Generation, although collectively, many of us undertook this process of reevaluation. The graduation speech that Steve Jobs, CEO and founder of Apple, gave at Stanford University in 2005 as he faced his own death is also illustrative of this sensibility and is worth noting here:

> Remembering that I'll be dead soon is the most important tool I've ever encountered to help me make the big choices in life. Because almost everything—all external expectations, all pride, all fear of embarrassment

or failure—these things just fall away in the face of death, leaving only what is truly important. Remembering that you are going to die is the best way I know to avoid the trap of thinking you have something to lose. You are already naked. There is no reason not to follow your heart.

For the men of the AIDS Generation, this ongoing evaluation of life and life choices is very present in their voices. A lifetime of expecting death has engrained this approach to living deeply into the consciousness of the men with whom I spoke and is not lost despite our advances in treating and maintaining the disease. This life lesson resounds deeply for each of them. In Project Gold, a 53-year-old African American man who was diagnosed in 1986 even suggested that contracting the virus in some ways saved his life by forcing him to confront his life and behavior, reexamine what truly matters, and appreciate his life as an older man:

> I love every gray hair I got, every wrinkle I got. I—I lve it. [Perry: Uh huh.] You know? I because of this virus now you know, um, I'm, um, more in tune with, you know, with, I'm more in tune with my body, you know, I'm—I'm just—just so careful about that. My health period so that's something—something to be thankful for. You know that's the only thing I can be thankful for for getting this virus [Perry: Uh huh.] is that it made me more aware; it made me just want to live harder, you know.

And another of the men from Project Gold, a 57-year-old mixed-race man diagnosed in 1987, expressed how HIV forced him to reevaluate as follows: "It's [HIV] made me a better person in the sense that I know that I'm living with something that's killing me and I want to live."

Living Longer

Part of making sense of getting older is the realization of and acceptance of a "normal" life expectancy after years of preparing for an early termination. Jokingly, Christopher, who seroconverted in the early 1990s, described it as follows: "Plus your doctor says, 'You'll likely now live to be 70, 75, and you'll probably die from something else.' " Although Christopher shared that idea with humor, there is much truth to it. A 52-year-old African American participant in Project Gold who has been living with HIV since 1987 shared a similar thought:

> It's—it's just a—the fact of understanding and knowing that I'm getting older and there's nothing that I can do about that and as long as I continue

to do the right things and take care of my health, I'll be able to live a lot longer. . . . I'm—I'm gonna die from old age and if the clubs are still open, you'll find me in a wheelchair sittin' in front of 'em.

Certainly a normal life expectancy is evident among those newly diagnosed who access and adhere to their treatments, as noted in a study of HIV-positive men conducted in Great Britain (Nakagawa et al., 2012). Although the men of the AIDS Generation did not have the luxury of early detection and treatment, their life expectancies are also likely somewhat "normal" if they follow the same course of care to all aspects of their well-being. In fact, according to this most recent study, the life expectancy is 75 years if HIV is diagnosed early, compared with 82 years for individuals without HIV; if HIV is detected late, the life expectancy of those with HIV is estimated at 71.5 years.

It is this matter of a normal life expectancy that most confused the men with whom I spoke. In Chapter 4, I proposed a set of actions that I believe explain the survival of each of these men, and their words and actions support these propositions. But logic and reason set aside, the men also expressed a more affective response to the explanation of their survival—that of luck. This idea appears earlier in the utterances of both Jackson and Bobby as they reflected on the concept of survivor's guilt and emerged again as Ryan, who is the youngest of the men at age 40, tried to make sense of his life as on older man:

The goal is just to get as much good and healthy time out of this life as possible. My mom is being treated for multiple myeloma and has had two stem cell transplants—currently undergoing chemo to—I am paraphrasing, but her doctors told her that there is never a "cure" but to get as many healthy years as possible, extending her life. That may be a long way off, but it is something that she always carries with her. The longer I live, the more I believe in the "just dumb luck" that comes our way.

Exhaustion and Trauma

For the last 10 years, I have mused on the aging of my generation of gay men. How would all of us emerge into this period of our lives when so many of those we loved had been defeated by AIDS, even as so many others somehow survived, but when all of us knew that one wrong decision could make us victims of this deadly disease? We all navigated the last 30 years of our lives step by step as if walking through a minefield, where with one wrong move, life could become forever altered. That is to say, collectively, the men of the AIDS Generation are traumatized from a lifetime of combatting AIDS and to some extent the sexual, physical, verbal, and emotional abuse many experienced as children due to sexual orientation. As previously noted, we have documented rates of posttraumatic stress disorder (PTSD) among older HIV-positive men as comparable to and surpassing those who have experienced specific traumatic events such as 9/11 (Halkitis, Kupprat, et al., 2013). Moreover, these elevated levels of trauma are not confined to gay men or simply those of the AIDS Generation but also include other groups such as HIV-positive women, who demonstrate PTSD rates five times higher than national samples of women (Machtinger, Wilson, Haberer, & Weiss, 2012). In a recent interview (Bernstein, 2013), the psychologist Walt Odets described, this condition and with regard to spencer Cox, as follows:

> It was an extraordinary trauma comparable to a wartime experience....For many gay men, after the epidemic was over, there was a loss of energy and vitality. It's like going from a car that runs on rocket fuel to one that runs on gasoline. And it had to be bewildering for Spencer.

Although Odets refused to use the term "posttraumatic stress disorder" in this interview, what he described is replete with the essence of PTSD.

During one portion of the focus group, several of the men engaged with Richard's story about preparing to die only to live. Although this was not the case for all of the men, it was true for a subset of them either because of their own experience or because of what they had witnessed in their social circles. This interaction, as shown to follow, is illustrative of the manner in which the men of the AIDS Generation are trying to make sense of their lives as older adults. There is no doubt that all are thankful to be alive, but this path and this reality is one that is fraught with decisions made during a lifetime when imminent death was never an abstract condition but an ever-present possibility/reality, which creates high levels of emotion burden:

RICHARD: I was as sick as you were talking about. It was when I started keeping my online diary. And I didn't say it at the time but I was really keeping the diary of someone who was dying. And—but you don't say that out loud to yourself. You don't say, "Okay, now I'm gonna be dead now in a couple of months." But I got so close and I was completely skull faced, completely bones and skeleton. And I stopped processing foods altogether. It was just really horrible. When I was finally on what they said was my deathbed, I had this strange uplifting feeling of like yes! Now I can just let go. I actually felt this great relief. And it was—it sort of blindsided me at the time. It was like oh good, the angel's gonna come and I'm just gonna get the fuck out of here. You know I was almost grateful. And then when the Crixivan lottery hit and I—you know 2 weeks later I stopped having diarrhea and started to come back to life. Then I had the great moment of now what the fuck do I do?

KERRY: I'm still there!

RICHARD: I was so—yeah. I was just so—I wrote a song about that too, by the way, called "Lazarus." You know, like I was almost grateful for the relief and then like the curtain was coming down, and it was fine. And then all of a sudden, curtain going back up again! Shit, now I gotta long road ahead of me and life started to seem like—

KERRY: What am I going to do for an encore, right?

BOBBY: I have to pay off those credit cards I ran up. [People laughing] You know?

RALPH: You just had an intermission is all you had!

In truth, the gay men of my generation, the AIDS Generation—all of us, HIV-positive or negative, across every race, ethnicity, and culture, from every part of our country, from stock broker to dancer to salesman—were robbed of a life filled with youthful frivolity, with endless optimism and hope. And as middle-aged men, we are as a group traumatized and fatigued from 30 years of war. Kerry feels this sense very deeply and he shared it in our group gathering:

> We are exhausted! And well before our time. [Eddie: Yes, yes.] And I think that's part of the problem too. [Eddie: Very much so.] I mean you talk about seeing death and getting used to it, but we were doing it in the 20s and 30s. It's normal to see it when you're 70, 50, 60. That's when it's normal. It wasn't normal for us. We didn't travel a normal route. And it's an exclusive kind of a club; that's why I love this thing.

Hope

The men who are portrayed in this work are men of my generation. Some are several years younger than me, like Ryan and Christopher; most are a few years older; and Eddie and Kerry, like me, will turn 50 around the time this book is published. There are no fixed rigid dates that define the men of the AIDS Generation; it is more a state of being. I have never been a particularly big fan of the rigid demarcation. For example, every website I read insists I am a member of the "baby boomer" generation because I was born between 1946 and 1964—1963 to be exact. I can tell you I feel no emotional or social connection to individuals who identify with that socio-generational group. The point here is that the men of the AIDS Generation are all hovering around middle age—some are in their early 40s and others are years beyond—and what binds us is our exposure to this pathogen during the formative years of our lives and ultimately our decades of fighting this viral enemy.

I could go on to suggest that 1996 marks an end date to the AIDS Generation. This marker does hold some significance. It is the year that the course of the AIDS epidemic in the United States was radically altered, and when so many who had little hope experienced a type of "resurrection," which has been documented in the literature as "Lazarus syndrome" (Adhiyaman, Adhiyaman, & Sundaram, 2007). (Richard's story noted previously is one such example of Lazarus syndrome.) It marked a turning point for all of the men I interviewed and for the entire gay population of the United States. So, with that in mind, perhaps there actually is a demarcation of 1996 for the AIDS Generation, but what binds us is less defined by this date than by our collective experience facing AIDS. This idea becomes illuminated when considering both Ryan and Christopher, who were the youngest men with whom I spoke, but who expressed feelings of connectedness more with older men who were also HIV positive and seroconverted before 1996 than with those of their age range who seroconverted at a later stage of life. I make these statements with complete knowledge that as a population we continue to be bombarded by this disease. Fortunately, those younger than us who are also living and affected by this disease are doing so in a time of greater hope.

For the men of the AIDS Generation, this current historic time period is also a time of hope. Having survived the darkest days of the epidemic, all 15 men with whom I spoke hover around middle age, a period of life that none truly expected to experience. Although this condition is one that the men accept and embrace, it is also one they must come to understand because for so many, life as an older adult was not a reality they had envisioned or imagined. John described it as follows:

I think that it's even gotten so bad now that I think about 8 years ago, I had a mental flip and now I'm convinced I'm gonna outlive everyone. I mean I just think the total opposite now. It's like, everyone's gonna be dead and I'm still gonna be going and I'm gonna be really lonely.

And Hal, who is married to his childhood sweetheart who is HIV negative, shared similar thoughts:

> My partner, we got life insurance for him because he's 52 and he could go before me. And I never thought I'd ever be in this position where I think, oh wow, I may outlive—because of this and because I have and because of all I do to sustain my well-being—I may outlive a lot of people that I didn't expect to outlive. What do you do with that?

This sense of optimism and hope also emerged in our pilot work and was framed by one of the men, a 54-year-old Project Gold participant who had been living with HIV since 1986, as follows:

> When you get older you realize that you gotta keep dreaming. You gotta come—when you achieve one dream, you gotta keep coming—coming up with new dreams and new dreams and new dreams. And keep constantly—keep dreaming.

Frustration

Many of the men of the AIDS Generation made life decisions based on an expectation that they would live 2, perhaps 5, maybe 10 years. Some spent their life savings, others abandoned their careers, and yet others enjoyed the escape of sex and drugs to numb the pain, loss, and fear they were experiencing. As a result, some of the men of the AIDS Generation find themselves at middle age with a possible life expectancy of 20 or more years and with an attempt to reinvent themselves, renegotiate the psychosocial struggles of previous developmental periods, and simply make sense of their lives. This struggle toward reconciliation and meaning making was most evident in Kerry's story. For Kerry, whose career was derailed by his HIV status, his emergence into middle age is fraught with physical conditions (described further later) but also with the frustration of trying to make and find his place in the world: "But at 50, when you've lost 20 years of your life, how do you get older and go back to business? You don't."

This situation is complicated for Kerry as he, like all the men of the AIDS Generation, remains dependent on his antiviral treatment, his health care, and his access to health services, which in his case would be undermined if he were to kick-start his career. Thus, for Kerry, his career has become maintaining his health, in the absence of any other meaningful work, and this is how he makes sense of his life as an older HIV-positive man:

> If I go back to business I lose my benefits. I lose my benefits; I lose 26 pills a day. I'm fucked. I'm back to square one. So everything I worked for in the '80s to get myself here to a place where I can at least have the medications and things that I need to survive, you know I can't ditch that. And I'm not going to. I don't plan on ditching it. And that, to me, is like a bigger job than anything else. You know?

A New Set of Deaths

For some of the men of the AIDS Generation, the reconciliation and understanding of the aging process is examined through the lens of an aging cohort of peers who, despite not being HIV-positive, are beginning to struggle with their own mortality. Issues of mortality also extend beyond the HIV epidemic as the men of the AIDS Generation grapple to understand why they have survived while others have perished at the hands of not only this dreadful disease but also other circumstances. During the gathering of the men, Christopher described one such experience and framed his understanding of the fragility of all humans:

> No, I just find as like, as I get older, like I—I never thought I'd live to be 30 and I watched a bunch of people I knew die from HIV and AIDS and whatnot. And I remember—I think I told you this in the interview that I had to tell an old boyfriend that I was positive because I think it was the right thing to do and I wanted to do it. And I told him. And I never in my wildest dreams ever thought that I would go to his funeral. I mean he was like killed on 9/11. You know, it's like the most random thing ever, and as I get older, I go to funerals now for people that—one of my friends just died last summer. I don't know, out of nowhere for no apparent reason other than heart failure, just died. And as I get older I think, well you know it's not just HIV now; it's other stuff. We don't all live forever.

This voice of survival in the midst of loss also came through from Hal, as he witnessed death throughout the course of his life from HIV but also from myriad other conditions, a life experience that empowered him to prepare for his own death. However, he also grapples with making sense of his own aging, what he values, and what the next decade of his life will bring:

When I was growing up, my grandmother killed herself when I was 7 and my mother killed herself when I was 10. My mother's younger brother killed himself when I was 13. My best friend fell out of a tree and broke his neck and died. My girlfriend—I mean it was like death was in my face relentlessly from the time I was a small child. And I knew about mortality. I knew what death was. I went fishing and hunting and I killed things; I saw how they died. So it wasn't such a mystery to me. The thing I didn't want to do was do it. It's like Woody Allen says he's not afraid of death. He just doesn't want to be there when it happens. And that was my feeling about all of it and I think that drove me too. There was this part of me that just felt like I'm gonna put this off.

And I lived in fear of dying throughout my entire diagnosis. Every day I would wake up and the first thing I would think is today gonna be the infection that's gonna get me? And what's amazing to me now is that at the age of 51 I think what am I gonna look like at 60? Will men still want me? It's like these are the kinds of questions I ask myself now. It's very possible my life will go on because I've just gone on.

In the end, all of the men of the AIDS Generation are grappling with how to understand the aging process and where life will take them next. This is a real, active, and conscious process for making sense of their lives that also leads to much confusion. Part of making sense of one's life is taking each day as it comes, as a gift after a lifetime of loss and despair, summarized perfectly in the words of Antoine:

You know, I mean we all had thing. I'll never forget, when the Golden Girls, first Ed, and the last five of us, that was our dream, to get old and live together. And I'm the only one here with Bianca, and it's like, "Okay, what do you want to do?" And now it's like I tell people, I go like this, and wherever the wind blows, that's where I'm going to be.

The Physical Deterioration

When I asked Gianni to describe how he feels as he is getting older and has lived with HIV for close to 30 years, he said:

All I know is that it takes a lot longer to heal. Like my back. When I used to pull it, it'd be fine in a day. Now it's 5 days—and cuts and colds. That's the problem of getting older. Or maybe it's because I'm poz. I dunno.

In this powerful verbal nugget, Gianni captures with pinpoint precision the complexities of aging with HIV. For all individuals the aging process generates physical manifestations that have not been previously experienced in one's life. This is the natural course of human development. But for the men of the AIDS Generation who have been monitoring their health closely for 30 years, it is unclear if these new and emerging conditions are due to aging, their HIV serostatus, or some interaction of both, thus creating an even greater sense of confusion and dread.

Here is what we do know. As of 2007, 22% of individuals living with HIV in the United States were ages 50 and older, with men who have sex with men (MSM) constituting approximately 50% of this population (Centers for Disease Control and Prevention [CDC], 2013a). Between 2007 and 2009, the number of adults ages 50 and over living with HIV increased from 209,433 to 256,259, and in 2009 85% of these were ages 50 to 59. By 2015, more than half of all those living with HIV in the United States are expected to have entered middle age (ages 50 or older) (CDC, 2013b; Gay Men's Health Crisis, 2010; Myers, 2009). This increase in prevalence of older HIV-positive adults is noted across the United States and in all 46 states with confidential HIV names reporting (CDC, 2013b). The cumulative effects of long-term survival due to antiretroviral therapy (ART; Palella et al., 1998, 2006) have resulted in part to the steep increase in the population of aging HIV-positive gay men.

For all HIV-positive individuals, the aging process is accelerated and confounded by chronic conditions that produce inflammation (Tien et al., 2010) as well as numerous other HIV-associated medical complications, including neurological abnormalities and cognitive deficits, all of which are associated with depression (Kohli et al., 2006). Older HIV-positive individuals have an increased likelihood of HIV- and non-HIV-related medical conditions. Moreover, health complications can be exacerbated by the long-term use of ART (Carr, 2000; Carr & Cooper, 2000). The biological process of aging itself, and the attendant loss of proper immune functioning, coupled with long-term immune activation due to ART use increases the risk for HIV-associated non-AIDS outcomes, including cerebrovascular and cardiovascular disease (Bozzette, 2011); osteoporosis and bone loss (Cotter & Mallon, 2011); kidney (Medapalli et al., 2012), liver (Vallet-Pichard, Mallet, & Pol, 2012), and lung disease (Crothers et al., 2011); and non-HIV-related cancers (Dubrow, Silverberg, Park, Crothers, & Justice, 2012), as well as severe hypogonadism (Cotter & Powderly, 2011).

Research also suggests that older age and HIV are independent risk factors for HIV-associated neurocognitive deficits (e.g., attention and working memory, executive functioning, etc.; Boissé, Gill, & Power, 2008; Brand & Markowitsch, 2010; Woods, Moore, Weber, & Grant, 2009). Although the severity of these deficits ranges from mild to moderate, their impact on activities of daily functioning, such as ART adherence (Zogg, Woods, Sauceda, Wiebe, & Simoni, 2012), medical management of multiple comorbidities (Cook, Sousa, Matthews, Meek, & Kwong, 2011), and other behavioral risk factors such as sexual decision making (Slavin et al., 2011), may be substantial. In addition, HIV infection among older adults is associated with elevated rates of psychiatric disorders such as anxiety, depression, and mood and substance use disorders (Horberg et al., 2008; Paterson et al., 2000).

These are the facts of aging with HIV, the conditions that the men of the AIDS Generation must face. My colleague Tony Urbina and I spoke about this matter a few years ago. His approach as an HIV care practitioner is to be proactive and treat his patients who were 40 or 50 with approaches that might be used for older adults not living with HIV. The goal is to provide care that prevents the onset of the conditions of aging such as hypertension, elevated levels of bad cholesterol, low testosterone, and diabetes. This is how Gianni describes the situation:

> Yeah I take my HIV meds—but only two of them. But I also take Lipitor, and Prilosec and Avapro, and now I also take supplements like tumeric to reduce inflammation. Yeah it's a lot of pills again, like the old days of treatment. Oh and I use the testosterone cream too.

Throughout our conversation, Kerry, more than any of the other men, attended to these physical manifestations, noting both his limited energy, likely due in part to hypogonadism, and his neurocognitive deficits, of which his is keenly aware: "And I—I don't have the energy. And I have—my—my memory's affected." Throughout our conversation, Kerry often expressed frustration as he described how he struggles with his executive function, particularly his working memory:

> I find it frus—I—I—I get it. I mean I find it frustrating when I know that I know—like I see something and it reminds me of something and I can't remember what the hell it is and I'm trying to remember. And it kills me.

In fact, he comes to understand this aspect of his physical being as a limitation that prevents him from truly meaningful work and parallels his experiences to others who are much older than he. Kerry spends a few hours of his time working in an office and describes this aspect of his life and well-being as follows:

> I go to this office and I help out once in a while when someone's out sick or something. There's a big family, it's a place I used to work, so I'll go there once in a while and work a week if someone goes on vacation. I can't—I can't keep up. There's a guy there who's 82. It's the—the owner's father does the collections. And he and I are on the same exact path and we get along like, you know, two peas in a pod. Because his memory's the same way mine is. He's able to do the same things I can, you know. And they have him on collections just to have him there to keep him active. And they let me come in just to keep me active—sort of thing.

And, after only a slight interjection by me stating "Right," Kerry exemplifies the condition he is describing: "And see, I totally forgot where I was going with that whole point." At this point I tried to assist Kerry and said, "You're—no, you're totally on track with the neurocognitive stuff. You were giving that as an example," at which point Kerry replied:

> The 82-year-old, but there was something to it. Something else. Maybe that was it. Maybe that was all the point. But see, like that happens. That never used to happen to me. I'm a sharp guy, like I'm not an idiot. That's the other thing. I'm smart, but I'm dumb.

As is so clearly evidenced in the story of Kerry, his struggle with his memory that he attributes to his HIV status does represent a physical deterioration, but it is also debilitating to him emotionally and socially.

Others, like Gianni, also expressed concern with the physical manifestations of the aging process, but in Gianni's case, the concerns were framed around truly becoming ill because of his age and more so due to his age and living with HIV:

> You know I'm older now. I know things happen, and I know they happen more to guys like me who are poz. So like the last year or so, I've been super aware of my body—like every little mark. I'm not sure why I'm doing it. Maybe I should stop reading all that stuff, like all the anal cancer stuff that is freaking me out.

The issue of anal cancer is one of particularly high significance to HIV-positive men, and one that I and my colleagues at the Center for Health,

Identity, Behavior and Prevention Studies (CHIBPS) have considered and shared with the gay community of New York City (Halkitis & Blachman-Forshay, 2011; Perez Figueroa & Halkitis, 2012). As is noted in these articles, exposure to at least two forms of human papillomavirus (HPV), 16 and 18, are linked to the development of cervical cancer and anal cancer, especially as seen in gay men. However, these conditions are more pronounced for HIV-positive men, as noted in the extraordinary and significant work of medical researchers like Stephen Goldstone, and could be of even greater significance for aging HIV-positive men, like those of the AIDS Generation (Goldstone, 2005; Palefsky, 2005). However, for many HIV-positive men the conditions that may lead to the development of anal cancer (i.e., high-grade lesions) remain unchecked by many heath care providers and could be detected early with a Pap smear. Stephen Goldstone, who is a dear colleague, often shares his dismay at the number of cases of anal cancer he detects that likely could have been prevented if appropriate screenings had been undertaken by primary care providers. For the men of the AIDS Generation, anal cancer is but one of the types of cancers, including lymphomas and malignancies (Hsiao et al., 2009) and prostate cancer (Crum, Spencer, & Amling, 2004), that may be more pronounced as they enter middle age.

The physical manifestations and complications of aging with HIV are abundant. Many of the men with whom I spoke shared these concerns. Ralph, who spent many years working as a bartender on Castro Street in San Francisco, was clear in his articulation of what so many face as they age—the expectation that the other shoe will drop. Perhaps this is a learned state after having witnessed death for 20 years, or perhaps it is because of information overload. Whatever the cause may be, many of the men describe an ongoing vigilance about their physical health, especially now as they are older:

> I remember when I was a kid I had ideas. Back then, some of them were silly but I was young. And I would think if only I could go to the next Ricky Lee Jones show and then wait for the next one. But then eventually I didn't even know when the next song was coming out. So apparently it wasn't the Ricky Lee Jones album that was keeping me alive, but I think it was just common sense. You know, I may be HIV positive, but also I have to worry about other things that will kill me. So basically I have to look both ways before I cross; I just don't want to get hit by a bus. There's more to worry about than HIV, I guess, especially when we're this age.

Despite this vigilance or hypervigilance regarding HIV and aging, there is and continues to be an optimism among these brave but battle-weary soldiers, an optimism similar to that which emerged even immediately after their diagnosis—a will to live and survive. In the world of Richard, the voice that emerges is that undeniable desire to live, which helps him confront the multitude of conditions he experiences:

> But sometimes it's hard because my thyroid's out; I've got diabetes, high blood pressure. I've got all that other stuff that you were talking about. My digestive system stopped working at one point and it finally got working again. It just seems like—there's a song in my show called "Friendly Fire"; the medications feel worse than the disease. Or is the disease worse than the medication? It's hard to tell because we take these things and each one is like a little poison dart that keeps us alive but also poisons us in a certain way.

The Physical Ravages of AIDS

Like all survivors of arduous battles, long-term survivors of AIDS bear their own physical battle scars. Besides the daily maintenance of HIV and precautions taken to avert the onset of other health conditions, some of the men of the AIDS Generation have visible markings of a life of HIV. These physical manifestations mainly are due to lipodystrophy (Carr, 2003), redistribution of body fat, with the most evident signs being sunken cheeks and a distended belly. Sunken cheeks are not uncommon for individuals as they age but are more pronounced among the HIV positive, especially older HIV-positive individuals who were prescribed certain classes of HIV treatments and particular medications early in the implementation of ART (Department of Health and Human Services, 2005, p. 1):

> Early studies suggested that lipodystrophy was associated with the use of protease inhibitors (PIs), a class of commonly prescribed anti-HIV drugs. However, other studies have shown that lipodystrophy also occurs in people who have never taken PIs. Evidence now suggests that lipodystrophy is linked to taking nucleoside reverse transcriptase inhibitors (NRTIs) and PIs at the same time.

As I looked around the room at the men of the AIDS Generation, some had clear indications of the condition and others did not, and some who likely had been afflicted with the condition were treating it with "fillers" such as

Radiesse® and Sculptra® injected into their faces. Patrick's voice was clear on this matter as he pursued treatment to confront this physical condition with little success:

> I worry abut my face too. I worry about—I've had the injections. I've had like 16 injections, 16 treatments. And it just keeps going down. And I'm at a point now where I say fuck it, I don't care.

Still, despite his inability to control the effects of lipodystrophy, Patrick has reached a sense of peace about this condition:

> You know, I've earned these. I've earned this face. And if people are gonna look at me weird about it, that's their deal. It's not my deal and I've been through a lot; they have no idea. And if there's judgment going on—yes, I was, I was judging them thinking they were judging me. And I'm really letting that go. And um, and [sighs] I've been through a lot and I deserve the good stuff that's coming. I deserve these wrinkles. I've earned these wrinkles. I've earned this face and that's my badge and I don't think I'm gonna have any treatments anymore.

Patrick seems to have channeled courage around his physical appearance, but my sense was that this was more bravado. Despite the men having managed to survive until middle age and to date contain the virus that afflicts them, the process of aging, and moreover aging as an HIV-positive gay man, is difficult. It is difficult physically as is shown previously, but it is also very difficult emotionally in the gay community, which is hyperattentive to looks and appearance.

In our communities, we have overdefined ourselves by our bodies and our appearance. Quite simply, you have the expected appearance and are "A-list" and noticed or you are not and you blend into the walls. Gianni experienced it as follows:

> For a good 20 years, I was at the center of this gay life in New York City. What [I] also did know was that I had a shelf life, and when I reached 40 I perceived my impeding expiration date. It is at that point that I removed myself from these social circles in fear of being one of those who blended into the walls and was unnoticed.

Perhaps for Gianni, the narcissistic break would have been too much for him to bear.

Often when I think of the expectations of appearance demanded by gay men—of hypermasculinity and physical prowess and beauty (Halkitis, Green, & Wilton, 2004)—I think of the work of Andrew Sullivan, which encapsulates this condition. In *Love Undetectable* (1999), Sullivan describes the circuit parties made legendary by the New York City bar the Saint and the men who navigated the contexts, underscoring the demand for physical perfection (p. 12):

> Begun in legendary disco in Manhattan, the Saint, they had mesmerized generation of homosexual urbanites. I was taken to one in the mid-1980s, as the plague began to descend, but even then its effects were hard to determine. What you saw was an oasis of astonishing masculine beauty, of a kind our society never self-consciously displays in the open. I remember feeling at first a gasp of disbelief, a sense that, finally, I was surrounded by visions that had only once existed in my head.

And within this spectacle of beauty and masculinity, there existed clear and defined rules for appearance that set those in the A-list apart from those who could not achieve the standard (pp. 12–13):

> While the slim and effeminate hovered at the margins, the center of the dance floor and the stage areas were dedicated to the most male archetypes, their muscles and arrogance like a magnet of self-contempt for the rest.

I too witnessed this spectacle, I too strove for the ultimate male archetype, and I too showed my disregard for those who did not meet the standards. Many of us did.

This is all to say that aging for any gay man is a complicated matter exacerbated by these expectations of the gay community—of hypermasculinity, beauty, and perfection. We may not like these values, but unless there is a major paradigm shift in what we value, this reality will exist in perpetuity.

It is in this context that the men of the AIDS Generation are aging. Managing their physical beings is complex due to the effects of aging and HIV, as well as the synergistic effects of aging with HIV. Add to the mix the expectations of our community and the demands for physical prowess and perfection, which are simply unachievable. For Ralph, who relied often on his appearance in his life, this situation is very pronounced and clear:

> All the time that we're watching our bodies, our physical bodies degenerate. I mean, no matter how happy you keep yourself. That's why it's hard to go

out these days because I find I try and compare myself to something that I've passed, as in my prime. So it's hard to go out and see people in their prime. That's kinda like their thing. I remember when it was mine, when I was in my prime too then.

Patrick's ideas also aligned with Ralph's. Arriving at this realization that he could not attain the stature required by the gay community because he is an older man managing HIV, Patrick sighed and said, "Oh I know. I look in the mirror every day and I still go 'god this is gross' but I'm gonna keep my body as well as I can but I'm not gonna do anything else. I need to try and make myself feel younger." The sentiment was shared by Eddie, who has come to accept the aging process and is making peace with his age and his body:

> It took me years to let my white hair grow out like this, I mean years, because trust me, if I would dye [my hair] and—oh, easily, it would be no problem to look like 30. Easily for me! Easily! I mean my body, I have a naturally sort of toned body. I mean, it's a blessing, but you know, I got tired of the dye and I got tired of just forgetting how old I said I was.

In the end, the process of aging for the men of the AIDS Generation will be fraught with many of the same medical sequelae facing all adults, as noted in the statement by a 57-year-old Project Gold participant:

> Getting older. This I—this is a hip replacement here. This one hurt me so bad, uh, last week I needed a cane to get around. The other hip. So, now it's time to have that done.

In truth, this could be any older man!

Getting Older in a Young Gay World

In the previous section, I considered the demands placed on gay men by their peers for physical perfection. This condition is one of which the men of the AIDS Generation are highly conscious and one of which they spoke abundantly during conversations. For many of these men, both the process of aging and combating HIV for decades create demanding realities, in part because of the expectations of physical perfection and in part because of our own youth-obsessed society, a condition that is also present in the gay population. This programming is also true for the men of the AIDS

Generation themselves. In fact, the extant literature has documented the difficulties experienced by some gay men in a youth-obsessed culture (see Gray & Dressel, 1985, for a review); however, as Gray and Dressel indicate, such conditions may not be confined solely to gay men but rather are pervasive conditions for all older individuals across sexual orientations. Still, for the men of the AIDS Generation, there exists the added burden of a ravaged body due to the inflammation and treatments of HIV, creating greater physical, social, and emotional challenges. Commenting on our obsession with youth, Ralph said, "While walking on the street—I'll admit it—I don't ever go, 'There's a hot old man.'" And when I shared with him my own removal from gay social venues at age 40, he simply added: "Well, you had to stop because you were kind of forced to. We're too old for that." Similarly, Christopher understood this idea of aging as follows:

> I think we just live as—America is just a youth-oriented society to begin with. So it makes it really hard to sort of navigate that. But I think, I find that gay men just tend to be—not unsupportive of each other, but I think they could be so much more supportive of each other. And it's kind of like when you're positive it's like, it's us and them; when you're older and younger, it's us and them. When you're richer and poorer, it's us and them. The Pines or Cherry Grove [two separate sections of the gay vacation destination in Fire Island, New York], it's us and them.

Still, for many of the men of the AIDS Generation, like Patrick, the aging process creates an emotional challenge for socialization in the gay community. Patrick encapsulates his feelings about getting older in a young gay man's world. Given my feelings about my own shelf life in the gay world, I completely understood Patrick's sentiments:

> That's the hardest thing for me, I think. That's the thing that—it's really hard. I'm in a relationship with someone that's a little bit younger than I am. I really enjoy my apartment. I like being home. I come home from work and I enjoy being home. I like being—I'm such a domestic now and I enjoy that. I've done the gay bar thing. I've done the circuit parties. I've done all that stuff. It just doesn't, you know?
>
> "Come on. It's good for you to go out!" So we went out, a couple of weeks ago we went out to a bar on 9th Avenue and said, you know, we did that a year ago and I hated it because I was just so—they're all so young—they're all so young. I was bitter; I'm a bitter old queen. And I thought, "Oh, this is terrible."

I've been seeing a therapist for a couple of years now and much better now. We went out a couple of weekends ago and he said, "So, this is good, right?" I said, "Yeah, it's fine." I'm out and I'm seeing them. They're still young and I'm enjoying my vodka and it's good. But you know what, I still don't—this isn't necessary for me. And I'm in a place in my life where I don't want to be reminded really of that. There are some men that love to see the youth; that—that revives them. And I'm not so much. I like to be around people my own age or around that proximity with similar experiences.

Tyronne, who was at the center of gay life working at the Saint as AIDS emerged, also understood the complexities of the aging process, the connection between his mind and his body, and a desire to keep his vitality in a youth-obsessed gay culture:

I don't think I can do some of the things I wanted to do as a gay man, like attract—like still attract guys like I used to—I mean I notice now—but that was one of the things why I really didn't want to get old was because I just still wanted to be same young person with the same—I didn't want my body to age because I felt like if my body aged then my mind would age too, and I would start living the way my body would, you know.

He then proceeded to describe his experiences as an aging gay man in relation to a younger generation, and the challenges that are evidenced even in attempting to role model for this new group of men:

The younger ones, I think they're not nice to the older gay men, but the older gay men are nice to the older gay ones. I see that a lot now, especially around the ages where I'm at, I guess maybe because we have a group, and we're always talking about how gay people need to start being a little bit more concerned for each other, a little bit more caring, you know, and not try to knock a girl down when she's—you know we're always trying to do something, so the older ones do, but not the younger ones so much, and they seem like they're hard to take advice, and to teach now.

A Yearning for the Past

Several years ago I was asked to write the foreword to my colleague Michael Shernoff's book, *Without Condoms*, which examines the practice of unsafe sex, barebacking, among gay men. Michael was a leader in the field of HIV prevention and care both in practice and in research. He too was a long-term survivor but died of AIDS complications in 2008 at age 57. In the foreword I state (p. xviii):

> I am reminded of the early days of AIDS, when community-driven efforts led by leaders such as Larry Kramer and Michael Hirsch and writers like Richard Goldstein and Robert Massa sought to unite us as a community in which the common enemy was the disease itself. I miss those days in which there was a zeitgeist that created a community of gay men united for a common cause and take offense to newer efforts, which in their attempts to unite serve rather to stigmatize, demonize, and alienate gay men rather than combating the disease itself.

Despite all the loss and death, there is a sentimental view of what had transpired in the first two decades of AIDS. As is noted in the previous extract, I too espouse such a sensibility. This nostalgic view of the past is shaped by what many of the men perceived as unification and solidarity in the gay community—a common cause against a common enemy—the HIV virus. This is certainly what is portrayed in my colleague David France's documentary *How to Survive a Plague*, even when the footage depicts bickering and disagreement at the ACT UP meetings. It is also how Kerry remembers those days. Reflecting on those ideas, Kerry said:

> I think it's just as tough to be an older gay man as it is to be a 13-year-old teenager who picks up all those magazines [referring to gay publications depicting physically idealized men]. I—I think the, um, I think the gay community came together in a way in the '80s like it never had before—but I see it as completely splintered now and I don't see any focus on anything anymore. And that saddens me a little bit. As an older gay man that saddens me. Because there is no history anymore. All of our history died. There's was—there's nothing—they don't have Michael Bennetts, they don't have, uh, I mean they don't have Halstons, they don't—they don't have those things—that we, you know—well, maybe not you, but that were a part of my life—part of everyone's life.

Perhaps more than for any other with whom I spoke, this yearning was most evident for Kerry, who asked, "Where do you go if you're an older gay positive man?" He recalls the days of support and socialization when gay men, and gay HIV-positive gay men, gathered:

> Well, I mean, are there even support groups? I looked into it. There aren't that many—there's not like a lot going on in terms of support groups. I thought those were wonderful and they never happened.

Recalling such gatherings, Kerry adds:

> Like Body Positive was great, but Body Positive is gone. Remember those dances? I never missed that dance. Never. I had a routine. I went—where did they have them? I don't even remember where they had them. . . . That's the last time I felt like any kind of a brotherhood with any kind of community.

And he mourns the loss of community as much as he mourns his losses from the epidemic:

> The loss and devastation was matched in slightly later years by the disbanding of the gay community. We got a pill. Stay away from them and you'll be fine. We totally left lesbians in the dust, just turned on them after they held our hands while we died. I do yearn for the community of the past in the very worst way and hope in my lifetime to see it again under much happier circumstances. I feel that I don't fit in anywhere in the gay community now. Then we were all one, accepting of each other, and that is no longer the case.

For Hal, there is also a sense of loss, but in his case, of the gay centers that permeated major cities like New York in the early days of gay liberation and prior to and during the early days of AIDS. In San Francisco this center was Castro, and in New York City this center was Christopher Street, a center that shifted to Chelsea after the epidemic emerged:

> I was walking up Christopher Street to my house today and had a moment of how gay it used to be hit me like a ton of bricks. I feel the same way about Chelsea. I miss all the fun we had.

Yearning, however, is not confined solely to the days of community organizing and social engagement. It is also connected to the reality of aging in a young gay man's world. As noted earlier, the expectations of physical prowess and perfection create demands for gay men that become unrealistic and unattainable as we mature and age. To this point, Ralph also expresses a yearning, but cast in the context of these realities and expectations:

> It seems there are plenty of single older gay men yearning for company and sitting lonely. We have the desire of sexual appetite but far less opportunities. Yearning becomes a way of life. It's sad to see and sad to be.

A New Generation of Gay Men Struggling With HIV

One voice that emerged often in my discussions with the men of the AIDS Generation concerned the ongoing HIV epidemic in gay men, especially in a new generation of gay men. This voice reflected many emotions including concern, confusion, and anger. At the same time, it ignited in many of the men a call to action to serve as role models and mentors to a new generation of gay men.

For many of the men, who were unaware of the consequences of their behaviors in the 1980s or who were infected even prior to the first signs of the epidemic in 1981, it seems inconceivable that a new generation of men would place themselves at risk given all of the knowledge we have developed regarding AIDS over the last 30 years. The whole idea of young men becoming infected in 2012 is anathema to many of them. It is in this portion of our discussion that I found myself most pushing back on the men's ideas and asking them to think beyond their own circumstances, to consider what it might mean be young and gay today, and why information might not be a sufficient protection. My conversation with Tyronne is illustrative of these interactions

PERRY: Let me ask you something else. I'm real interested to hear what your thoughts are on this. So when you look at HIV in like this city, and this country, like, so like—there's no doubt in my mind that gay men—like, we're like—maybe we're like 3% to 5% of the population, right, but we're like 55% to 60% of the epidemic, right, so like when you look at the patterns of who gets infected, you see young Black guys from 13 to 29 huge, the White guys are kind of even, and then the White guys in their 30s, pfft—through the roof. What do you think is going on with the young Black guys that they're getting infected at younger ages?

TYRONNE: I don't know. I mean, they're getting education because they're getting it from schools like—on the Internet, I really don't know. With all the education, and all of the medicines, and everything, like I don't understand why.

PERRY: Do you think the information is enough? Let me ask you it this way—because I do this game with myself all the time. Make believe—make believe we're 18 again. It's 2012, and we have really, really, really, really fabulous skin again, right, like 18-year-olds' skin, right, that we don't have to moisturize and shit, that takes like forever to take care of, do you think you would be safe all the time?

TYRONNE: Yeah.

PERRY: You do?

TYRONNE: Because the youth—

PERRY: You think you would be safe?

TYRONNE: The youth are irresponsible.

PERRY: You think you would be safe?

TYRONNE: If I knew what I did now way back, of course.

During the course of our conversations, I described to the men of the AIDS Generation my research program with young gay men, a cohort study in which we follow a group of approximately six hundred 18-year-old young men as they emerge into adulthood and assess patterns of risk and resilience and the factors that predispose these patterns. Participants meet with us every 6 months and are also tested for HIV infection via oral antibody testing. The project is called Project 18 (aka P18) (Halkitis, Moeller, et al., 2012), and as might be expected, a subset of the men seroconvert during the course of the study. When I shared this with Bobby, he found the situation incomprehensible given the social advances gay men have made:

Which is really horrifying to me that in a world where there are positive images finally of gay peop—of gayness for people to access it does get better. There's Dan Savage, there's Will and Grace, there is blah, blah, blah that these young minds aren't, you know, reaching out and grabbing on to what—I guess I feel it's the gay version of "Oh, when we were a kid we had to walk uphill both ways." They all have it so easy, go access, go—you can ask your boyfriends to the prom.

Similarly, Antoine, who lost almost all of his friends in the first two decades of AIDS, shared this voice of sadness about the behavior of younger gay men, especially given the information that is available to them:

It makes me sad. Because you're letting 8 minutes of pleasure take away your choice. And you don't have to because back in our time, we didn't know. We didn't know that a simple little rubber could be, could protect us from a lifelong disease.

For Hal, the new seroconversions are a source of great anger, which he attributes to the marketing of HIV treatments:

Oh, one of the things that irritates me so much is that young people are being seroconverted and I blame the drug companies and the ads for the drugs and the men were all smiling and I think these kids think that, "If I get infected I can just take the drugs." I think they have no idea of what kind of a commitment it is to take them, the side effects, that you're doing it for life, that you're gonna run into all sorts of other problems. That you're gonna shit your pants. You know, it's like they have no idea. They have no idea the kind of tenacity it takes to, for me, for 14 years to swallow these pills every day and then start to have to swallow Crestor and Lovaza and blood pressure medicine and all sorts of other things because of aging and because of genetics and God knows what else.

In the course of our conversation and when I pushed back, Hal came to understand the complexities that young gay men face. Still, his overriding belief was that young men simply no longer feared HIV because it is not their primary presenting problem:

> And I think with the young adults I think you're right about all those factors playing into it but I also think that there is this prevailing attitude that the epidemic is over. That HIV is a chronic manageable illness. And I think it gets pervade not just—not so much even in the media because I don't think there's that much attention on HIV and AIDS anymore.

This too was an understanding voiced by Andre, who expressed the uncertainty of life with HIV even in light of treatment advances: "So just because you can take a pill for one thing doesn't mean—and guess what, that pill's for the rest of your life. And we don't—still don't know the long-term effects." Finally, Hal spoke from a place of anger insomuch as the attitude toward HIV, which he believes permeates our society and which envisions AIDS as "cured," also affects him personally in how he speaks about his own condition:

> But a common response if I'm complaining about my health or anything going on is, "Well you have these drugs now. And you should be grateful. And look at all the life you have that you would—look at the 14 years you've had that you wouldn't have had." It's like it's constantly minimized. No one wants to say, "Oh this must suck for you to take pills and shit your pants for a year." Which I just went through with Viramune. I just changed my combination.

For subset of other men, like Gianni, there was a similar sentiment, although he had a more compassionate approach to the struggles young gay men currently face:

> Look, I didn't know there even was an HIV. It was 1981. No one knew. What if I was 18 now? These guys know what's going on. Would I always use condoms? I don't know. I'm not sure I would.

To address this concern about the new infections among young gay men, Bobby and his husband, John, speak publicly at schools and other gatherings of youth about their HIV status. Still, to this point, Bobby recognizes that even when he shares his story of struggle and near-death experiences due to AIDS, it is difficult for a new generation to fully understand the impact of the disease:

> To me I went and did an HIV talk out in Stonybrook and of course, we have all been through horrible things. I weighed 135 pounds and couldn't swallow my own spit. I've been in horrible physical condition. But I'm 47; I look better than I am. I'm built like I've never been built and things are really good. So where do you balance the story to these younger people and say, "Please don't get HIV; please don't go do that. But if you do, there's a lot of it's—." There's a lot of problem with that. You see what I'm saying? It's this weird, two parts of our story. I mean it sent me into a spiral of addiction and yet I'm happier and healthier and more secure than I've ever been in my life.

In this regard, Hal also describes the confusion that might be experienced by some who experience vibrant, healthy, older HIV-positive men. However, he notes that what they do not see is the struggle so many of the men of the AIDS Generation face to simply stay alive. During our focus group, Hal expressed these ideas clearly, which Eddie also acknowledged:

> I think it's also confusing to younger people too because we look good now. [Eddie: Yes.] They listen to us tell these stories and they're like, "But you look good." [Eddie: Right.] It's like they don't—right over their heads and the ads where everybody's for the drugs whatever and smiling and climbing mountains and having a great time, actually I've had diarrhea for a year. I've been shitting my pants for a year. That's what you get with these pills and it's like—but when I worked for GMHC, we did an outreach program, an education program and all the Broadway shows. And Starlight Express was one of them. And we got there and no one showed up. And the stage manager walked out and said, "They're 18 years old. They do back flips in 80-pound costumes and they don't think they're ever gonna die." [Eddie: Right.]

But to this point, Hal also recognizes that like these young men with whom he is speaking, he too espouses a sense of invincibility, one that perhaps explains his survival to this day:

> So it's like, and I remember being that age and thinking I'm never gonna die. It's in the back of your mind you know you're gonna, but it's like it's really not ever gonna happen to me.

And for Antoine, like Hal, Bobby, and John, there are ongoing efforts to protect these young men through their education and advocacy activities:

> And I'm not saying not to have sex. I'm just saying, you know because I, in fact when I leave here, I'm going to a group that I'm a mentor. It's called Royal Flush and Swag, where we mentor 18-year-olds to 25, and as I say to them, "Don't—forever's too long a period of time for you to give that away to somebody else. You know, when you get ready to have sex, you should have two condoms. One for you, and one for him. And if he doesn't have one in his pocket, ask him why." You know because even the guys that I sleep with, you know, I'll say to them, "Where's your condom?" You know, and if they don't have one, then I'm like, "What made you think we were going to do this without it?"

It is clear in these voices that we, the men of the AIDS Generation, those who have survived, both positive and negative, are now the elder statesmen. Despite the fact that so many of us have died and there is a huge hole evident in our generation, there is a commitment to protect the future generations of gay men from this disease. But I wonder if our approach is correct? Are we too HIV centric at a time when HIV is not the same primary presenting problem it was for us? In this regard, Christopher noted, "I think it's not the same. A diagnosis of being HIV positive is—isn't the same diagnosis it was 20 years ago, or even 15 years ago." And differentiating experiences for a new generation of gay men from his own life experiences, Christopher added:

> I think for a lot of people, it just—they're either able to incorporate it in their life, or rate it in their life, or they get involved in a support group or something, they get the information and the resources they need and like they can already like forget it. I don't think—I mean, I—I don't survey people, it's just my—my guess that people just—there's not an urgency anymore and people probably talk in their own circles.

I too believe this issue of urgency is key in understating how we work with a new generation of gay men around the issue of sexual safety and HIV.

Over the last several years, I have spoken about the needs of younger gay men and called for a holistic approach to their care, a reframing of our HIV prevention efforts where we move beyond the virus and consider all aspects of health, including the social and emotional aspects of well-being (Halkitis, 2010a; Halkitis, 2012a). I also have argued that despite our best attempts, discrimination and homophobia are very present in the lives of young gay men, that these social conditions place them at risk for HIV and other health disparities (Halkitis, 2011), and that ultimately if we are to effectively combat HIV in gay men, we simultaneously must fight these conditions. It is why I have written about President Obama's support of marriage equality as protective of gay men's health (Halkitis, 2012b). It is why I believe enacting legislation and protecting our civil rights are the best solutions to the HIV epidemic in gay men. Treating young gay men with respect is also evident in our national HIV strategy, which articulates this holistic approach to HIV prevention. Condoms and safe sex strategies work, but they are behavioral patches to the much bigger problem—that of discrimination and homophobia—that perpetuate this disease in our population. My colleagues at GMHC have stated this eloquently as one of their HIV prevention approaches for gay men, calling for social marketing that increases family acceptance and reduces antigay stigma (Cahill & Valadéz, 2012). Richard also understood and espoused this notion that discrimination fuels the HIV epidemic in young men and has directed his efforts, in part, to helping young gay men navigate their places in the world:

> And I—and you know, I realized that perhaps [the musical I wrote], doing my online diary, all of those things were—were just survival instinct for me. But I realize that I put myself in the position of where, um, people look up to me. Young people—I get e-mails from young people all the time. I'm on the board of directors of Youth Guardian Services, which is an Internet peer group support group, uh, where we—we've created, um, e-mail lists limited—that are age limited. So 18 to 21, 21 to 25, 13 to 18. And only kids of those ages can be on those lists. Not even, um—even—even the people monitoring the lists are of that age. And so this was started by a 19-year-old who I met online, and I was giving him advice, and he was giving people advice at the age of 19. And so, um—so I've been actively involved in, uh, supporting young people and, uh, with PFLAG [Parents, Families, and Friends of Lesbians and Gays]. I do concerts for PFLAG. We're about to do a new program called Out of the—Out of the Silence. And it's a, uh, telegraphic exhibit that's going to travel that, uh, has quotes from young people who are coming out of the closet and—and bullied and all of that. And my big piece called New World Waking, two of the songs are based specifically on two kids that were bullied and what their mothers did and how their mothers reacted.

With Richard's voice we return again to the idea of legacy but also see how this legacy is being transmitted to help protect a new group of young men who are emerging into adulthood with HIV still omnipresent in their lives and in all of our lives. This voice also emerged from Andre as he described the ongoing challenges of being gay:

> There's still a struggle to some—I mean, just because you can be out in a crowd doesn't mean it's easy. You still have to face those people at school who just don't get it. You know, family may be accepting, but there's always something. There's—there's a dig, there's a word, there's a comment somewhere. You know, we love you, but—or someone had a sign at Folsom. They were on the high line and they had a sign. It was a religious sign. It was like, "You gays are going to hell," or something like that.

And in my conversation with Christopher, as we discussed the lives of young gay men, he too noted the ongoing struggle these men likely face with their sexuality that places them at risk for HIV and other health conditions, which starts with an inability of some, if not many, families to negotiate an understanding of the same-sex desires of their children:

> Um, I think with all the resources out there it should be less [HIV], but I think—I think people like read the materials or get the information, they probably don't put it into action because I think—I still think people look at gay sex as being a secret. Or some element of it is a secret. You know, you're taking it up the ass, you know, you're asking for HIV. And I—I think—I think that gay men in general and people in general, families don't talk about sex in a healthy way. And I just think in the family setting, it's just uncomfortable.

In fact, Christopher raises a critical point regarding family acceptance supported by the literature. In a recent study by Ryan, Russell, Huebner, Diaz, and Sanchez (2010), the role of family acceptance was found to be critical in protecting against negative health outcomes. In the sample of 245 lesbian, gay, bisexual, and transgender (LGBT) adolescents and young adults, greater acceptance was predictive of greater levels of self-esteem, social support, and general health and protective against depression, substance abuse, and suicidal ideation and behaviors. One can easily translate this finding to protection for young gay men against HIV. Kerry spoke of such family support regarding his younger HIV-negative partner, whose mother openly discussed issues of sexuality and safer sex with her son:

> Um, he's very well—he—his mother worked at Kings Park Psychiatric Hospital and for some reason, I don't why, she was tied into the AIDS

thing very early on. Uh, maybe because they dealt with a lot of junkies and addicts and stuff like that. So he was—and he's 13 years younger than me. So he grew up with a knowledge—a working knowledge. Not like the kids today. He grew up with a working knowledge of AIDS, so he knew what was safe, what wasn't safe.

Yet even in these circumstances and social conditions that are not ideal for all youth in the sexual minority, Christopher also notes that as a society we are heading in a better direction—one that will likely improve the health of gay men and may in turn reduce the transmission of HIV:

> And I think—I think that it's just so ingrained in the gay culture that it's sex before dating, because we're not allowed—we weren't allowed—us grow-ing up, we weren't allowed to date. Gay men can date now as young people. And going back to telling an 18-year-old, I would say that. Date because you can. You know, go out because you can. Enjoy someone's company because you can. I'm not saying it's have it—or don't have sex with them, but you can have a good time without that.

In the end, however, many of the men expressed a compassion for a new generation of gay men and hope that the lives of these men will not be burdened, as were our lives, and that perhaps they could learn from our collective experience, a sentiment that Tyronne expressed as follows: "I'm hoping that they're gonna take something from the generation of us you know and take it with them." Collectively, they also believed that a new generation of gay men infected with the virus will also struggle with issues similar to those of the men of the AIDS Generation, although perhaps without the conditions of imminent death. During the focus group and to this point Christopher said, "I think it'll be more like people with a chronic illness like diabetes," to which Ralph quickly responded, "And they'll have to deal with being old." Yet collectively as a group, the men of the AIDS Generation believed that the circumstances for this younger group of men infected with HIV would be qualitatively different from their own due to treatment advances that will likely prevent the disease from derailing their lives:

> I think what we've had to deal with that they won't is—it's a major thing is some of us have had to, we had our life kind of what I was gonna do and then I hit this AIDS thing and my life went completely different and then I stalled my career somewhere. And now I'm to an extent I'm scrambling;

I'm like, what's next? And that's the thing that they're not gonna have to think about.

Kerry sighed and surmised perfectly, stating, "They don't have the horror. I mean, we lived through horror. These kids, they don't have that." And as group, we were all grateful that another generation of gay men will not have to witness and experience what we, the men of the AIDS Generation, collectively share. That said, we desperately want these younger men to learn from our life experiences.

Conclusions

By 2015, half of all Americans living with HIV will be age 50 and older. A substantial portion of these older HIV-positive individuals are gay men—gay men like those of the AIDS Generation who have entered or are about to emerge into middle age. "Yet the world is unprepared to deal with the aging population with HIV" (Mills, Bärnighausen, & Negin, 2012, p. 1270). For the men of the AIDS Generation, like all others who are also aging, this period of life is uncharted territory. However, what is different for these men is that this developmental stage of life comes after lifetimes of negotiating and managing their health and well-being in their battles against AIDS.

To date, we know little about the needs of an aging generation of baby boomers who for all intents and purposes will have differing expectations from previous generations (Healthcare Intelligence Network, 2006). Even less is known about those baby boomers who are gay, and we are only beginning to scratch the surface of our understanding of the needs of aging gay HIV-positive men (Halkitis, Kupprat, et al., 2013). Within the subset of these aging seropositive men are those who have been combating the virus their entire adult lives and for whom the physical, emotional, and social complications may be even more pronounced. Some policy makers, like Cahill and Valadez (2013), express great concern that our health care system is ill equipped to meet the needs of an aging generation of HIV-positive individuals. I am less concerned about this matter, given that many HIV-positive older individuals, like the men of the AIDS Generation, are empowered to control their heath considering the manner in which they have managed their health across their lifetimes. Nonetheless, the ideas shared by the men with whom I spoke indicate the complexity of this aging process including but not limited to understanding one's legacy, grappling to understand how one has survived the epidemic, and negotiating one's place in a gay culture where the burdens of age and HIV all but make the men of the AIDS Generation invisible.

Recently, in the United States, there has been increased attention on the health needs of lesbian, gay, bisexual, and transgender (LGBT) individuals. The care of LGBT individuals and of aging LGBT individuals is informed by the recent report of the Committee on Lesbian, Gay, Bisexual, and Transgender Health Issues and Research Gaps and Opportunities of the Institute of Medicine (2011), which has demonstrated the health disparities experienced by sexual and gender minority populations. Most current models of successful aging do not consider LGBT individuals, although recent efforts by Van Wagenen, Driskell, and Bradford (2013) have attempted to improve this knowledge base and suggest that surviving and thriving are critical to understanding the success of this segment of the population. This latter idea speaks to the realities of the men of the AIDS Generation in middle age.

Moreover, HIV is only one of the health disparities faced by gay men, which also include heightened levels of mental health disorders and substance abuse, as well as physical and emotional victimization (Halkitis, Wolitski, & Millett, 2013). These conditions transgress HIV status in both gay male and aging gay male populations. The tragic events leading to the death of a New City therapist, Bob Bergeron, a well-respected and well-known gay man approaching middle age who provided care for many seropositive men of our generation (Bernstein, 2012a), illuminates the complexities and demands placed by our own gay culture on our lives—that of physical perfection and beauty, which of course fades with age—ideas shared abundantly by the men of the AIDS Generation. Still, and regardless of the sources of our health burdens, attending to the needs of gay men broadly and aging gay men specifically is a matter of critical importance. To attend to these maters, Senator Michael Bennet of Colorado introduced a bill in 2012 that calls for increased federal support to older LGBT people through the Older Americans Act, which to date includes no mention of LGBT older adults (Espinoza, 2012); numerous groups, including the AIDS Community Research Initiative of America (ACRIA; Brennan-Ing & Tax, 2013), as well as Services and Advocacy for GLBT Elders (SAGE) and the Movement Advancement Project (MAP), which coauthored a report (SAGE & MAP, 2010), have been lobbying to have both older LGBT adults and olderHIV-positive adults designated as the populations of greatest social need.

Yet for the men of the AIDS Generation, being middle aged is a victory after a lifetime of battles. As they reexamine the earlier period of their lives while negotiating the issues of generativity and legacy, they have much to be proud of. This will to live and survive that permeated so much of their adult lives is also a critical element in preventing their middle ages from being defined by stagnation and despair. Despite the burdens faced by these men as they age, they enter this portion of their lives grateful to be viable and vibrant individuals. Their battle scars are evident on every level—physical, emotional, and social. But these battle scars define who they are, the power they have demonstrated to the world, and the resilience they have embodied and make them all the more beautiful, perhaps even more beautiful than a carefree, free-spirited young gay man of 20.

On May 9, 2013, I had the privilege of witnessing the beauty and power of hundreds of HIV long term survivors as I moderated the community forum, "Is This My Beautiful Life," held in New York City and organized by a group of us as the Medius Working Group, in honor of Spencer Cox. One month after that momentous event, the success and the challenges of the aging HIV-positive population finally received national attention, in John Leland's *New York Times* article (Leland, 2013).

CHAPTER 6 | Resilience

A Lifetime of Living With AIDS

If *Gone With the Wind* has a central theme, I suppose is the theme of
survival. What quality is it that makes some people able to survive
catastrophes and others, apparently just as brave and able and strong,
go under? I have always been interested in this particular quality
in people. We've all seen the same thing happen in the present
depression. It happens in every social upheaval, in wars, in panics, in
revolutions. It's happened all the way down history from the time the
barbarians sacked ancient Rome, And before that, I suppose, some
people survive disasters. Others do not.

—MARGARET MITCHELL, 1936,
FROM PUBLIC BROADCASTING SERVICE, 2012

Never, never, never, give up.

—HAL, 2012

IT IS DECEMBER 1, 2012, as I start this chapter, the 25th commemoration
of World AIDS Day. Much has transpired since the first World AIDS Day
in 1987 in terms of understanding, managing, and treating this disease. In
fact, television advertisements have been aired for the new at-home HIV
test. Still, in 2011, between 31 million and 36 million were living with
HIV worldwide, 2.5 million of whom were infected that year. And despite
the availability of effective treatments, 1.7 million individuals died of
AIDS complications in 2011, with 25 million deaths in the last 30 years,
according to the World Health Organization (2011). In the United States,
which has always been on the forefront in the fight against AIDS, some

40,000 to 50,000 new infections are detected annually (Centers for Disease Control and Prevention [CDC], 2012b), and gay men experience this health disparity more than any other group (CDC, 2012c), accounting for over 50% of all these infections, and over 60% in large urban areas like New York.

> The war against HIV/AIDS is far from over, U.S. health officials said on Thursday, with gay and bisexual men in urban centers accounting for most new infections in the United States. Nearly 29,000 new cases of HIV, the AIDS-causing virus, were attributed to gay and bisexual males in 2010, and 82 percent of those cases occurred in large cities, the U.S. Centers for Disease Control and Prevention reported. "The HIV epidemic in the United States highlights inequities," said Dr. Jonathan Mermin, director of CDC's Division of HIV/AIDS Prevention. "One is that gay and bisexual men are over 40 times more likely to have HIV than heterosexuals, and urban areas of the United States have higher HIV prevalence than rural areas." (Reinhberg, 2012)

It is within this context that the men of the AIDS Generation continue their lives and emerge into older age. A lifetime of surviving HIV is a sobering reality heightened by the perpetuation of the epidemic in our community and within a new generation of gay men (CDC, 2012c, 2012d). And the more things change in handling this disease, the more they stay the same in terms of where the epidemic resides. Thirty years after the initial detection of the disease, the gay population remains under attack by this virus.

Simultaneously, those living with HIV in the United States continue to age. The men of the AIDS Generation are very much a part of this aging cohort despite a lifetime of never expecting to reach middle age. Each of them has survived, and as has been described in the previous chapters, each of them grapples with the ongoing demands of HIV coupled with the social, emotional, and physical manifestations of an aging body. The men of the AIDS Generation, despite their multitudes of losses and the myriad challenges they have faced since young adulthood, have survived, confronting the new dilemmas created by middle age. Like the work of Margaret Mitchell, if there is a main theme that runs throughout this volume, it is that of survival, and as stated by Hal in the opening of this chapter, it is about never giving up.

What becomes clear in the stories of the men with whom I spoke is that these men—the men of the AIDS Generation—are all truly resilient. Hal described it as "extremely adaptable, sure footed" and extended his thinking by stating, "I believe in hoping, happy endings, triumphs." In concluding this volume, it is this question that I seek to explore: How do I come to understand the men of the AIDS Generation as resilient?

Focusing on Resilience

On December 9, 2012, I attended the 20th annual Research in Action Awards sponsored by the Treatment Action Group (TAG). This was a momentous occasion and an opportunity to spend time with those men of TAG, including Mark Harrington and Peter Staley, whom my partner Robert Massa held in such high admiration and esteem. It was also an opportunity to be in a room celebrating the resilience of our community in the fight against AIDS. Several were honored, including Dr. Francois Barre-Sinoussi, who was part of the Pasteur team which identified the HIV virus; Dr. Paul Farmer of Harvard; and science writer Jon Cohen. Among them also was the actress and activist Judith Light, who spoke eloquently and reminded us that at a time in the 1980s when the Reagan administration was all but ignoring us, we refused to lie down and die—that we refused to be victims and fought for our lives. I was also reminded of how my own city's mayor, Ed Koch, was intractable and weak in his response to the epidemic—a condition captured with power in Larry Kramer's *The Normal Heart* (2000) and an issue David France described with pitch perfection upon Koch's death in 2013, stating, "Koch's failure in AIDS should be recalled as the single-most significant aspect of his public life. The memories of all we've lost deserve no less." Having witnessed the AIDS crisis in my world as a young man in the 1980s and Koch's lack of care and concern and outright antipathy to the gay community, I think it is safe to say that Koch was indeed one of the great villains in our war against AIDS. Thus, as I heard Judith Light speak, her words and the manner in which she delivered them resonated perfectly with me as I thought of this volume, the men of the AIDS Generation, and my own life. And I thought of our resilience.

Referring to the ACT UP movement depicted in *How to Survive a Plague*, Jacob Bernstein (2012b) writes, "...to Mr. France's additional dismay, little credit had been given to the activists who worked tirelessly throughout the '80s and early '90s, in many cases laying down in the streets to try to bring attention and money to the disease." I agree with David wholeheartedly and take that idea one step further. Little credit is given to the gay men of the AIDS Generation, some of whom were activists, and all of whom have managed to live through the epidemic with dignity, all the time fighting for their lives, not only through activism but also through the maintenance of "normality" in their bodies, in their emotions, and in their relationships.

One can endlessly enumerate the difficulties of living with HIV. There is no denying that these circumstances have been challenging for the men with whom I spoke, and in fact for all men of our generation. I am reminded that all World War II Holocaust survivors are given their due credit and place in history—not just those who risked life and limb to save others—and rightly so. These incredible men and women need nothing more than their incredible feats of survival as their legacies, again rightly so. This should also be so for the men of the AIDS Generation.

Numerous behavioral and medical studies have examined and characterized the deleterious conditions of being infected with HIV (e.g., Heckman, Kochman, & Sikkema, 2002; Kirk & Goetz, 2009). Yet the voice of survival and resilience is one that is often lost in the conversation in terms of their lifetimes and specifically as they emerge into older adulthood as indicated by Emlet, Tozay, and Raveis (2011). Perhaps this is because we as scientists tend to focus on deficits and build our theories and interventions from that perspective. This deficit perspective is particularly evident in the literature on aging gay HIV-positive men (e.g., Grov, Golub, Parsons, Brennan, & Karpiak, 2010; King & Orel, 2012) that describes high levels of mental illness, stigmatization, and isolation in the absence of the resilience so many older HIV-positive gay men, and HIV-positive individuals more broadly, demonstrate. Perhaps it is about perspective, because only now is it becoming apparent that a generation of men, the AIDS Generation, have created lives and continue to live in manners from which we all can learn. Or perhaps it is because it is about timing, and therefore, developmentally this is the appropriate period for all of us to remember the conditions through which we have lived over the last several decades. And finally, perhaps, as I have explored in Chapter 5, it is about legacy—our individual and collective legacy as a generation of men and the homage we must pay to those we have lost, and as an affirmation of our lives, that may serve as a model for future generations of gay men.

Drawing on the data that have been examined throughout this book—the reactions and strategies that are described in the previous chapters—this chapter will synthesize the ideas that have been explored and examine how these strategies for survival can be understood in relation to paradigms of resilience. I will begin by examining how the men of the

AIDS Generation come to understand this concept of resilience and then inform the discussion with their life stories and the actions they undertook to survive that speak to this construct. Thereafter, I examine how the men of the AIDS Generation would advise a new generation of young gay men who, like themselves 20 or more years ago, are newly infected with HIV. This synthesis of ideas will then be considered in relation to a set of practical concrete suggestions for anyone living with HIV—suggestions that also may be applicable to others living with different yet equally challenging chronic health conditions. As has been my approach throughout this volume, I will consider resilience as it is evidenced in the physical, social, and emotional domains.

Defining Resilience

As part of our ongoing conversation, I asked the men of the AIDS Generation to describe how they make meaning of the construct of resilience. Most often they described resilience in relation to their own personal challenges managing HIV. This included the stress created by the disease and the steps they enacted to manage the health crises that emerged over the course of their adult lives. Richard expressed it as follows in relation to his near-death experience prior to 1996:

> Resilience means making the choice, after months and months of vomiting, diarrhea, and being in pain and finally crawling back out of the hole, only to find yourself once again attacked and struck down even further, to take the step-by-step push to get back on top, even though you know that, physically, the top of the mountain is not possible. But you strive on.

This understanding of resilience is also very evident in Richard's life as he ages and faces new health challenges, perhaps not as severe as what he experienced in the mid-1990s but as physically and emotionally painful: "For me, lately, it's been kidney stones. One hit after another, leaving me in tears of despair, losing the will to fight on. But then, working it through, sticking it out, and making myself endure." Christopher also understood his management of HIV and more importantly his survival with HIV as illustrative of resilience, as a man who soon will have lived more years as HIV positive than HIV-negative:

> When I was first diagnosed I never thought I'd live to be 30, let alone 40. My days with HIV, quickly turned into months, and then years and in another

2 years I'll have lived with having HIV longer than I lived without having HIV. At one of the first support groups I've ever attended, somebody said, "Right now, we aren't dying from HIV/AIDS; we're living with it." For me, being resilient had meant that I've learned to live my life with HIV and all the issues that come with it. I've learned how to navigate, medical and insurance red tape, hold down a job, a relationship of 22 years, and do what I can in terms of helping others who live with HIV. I'll never say it's been easy. I've dealt with everything from depression to sex addiction, but somehow I've managed to get up and move forward. I would never say I've returned to the previous state of normal functioning, but I feel like I did find a "new normal."

Similarly, Jackson also understood his management of the disease as well as his ability to return to a sense of normalcy after health and other associated challenges emerged as resilient. But for him, resilience was informed by his behaviors to learn all he could about HIV and through the activism in which he actively engaged:

To me, resilience is the ability to bounce back from difficulties. Initially, I think facing the shock of what was happening and realizing I was smack dab in the middle of the AIDS crisis sent me, not into despair, but into a realization that I was going to have to steel myself. I'm a natural researcher, so sorting through all the confusing information about AIDS and HIV, separating fact from fiction, energized me. At first I had to push myself to visit friends in hospitals, attend memorial services, and while I was telling myself I was being altruistic and benevolent while holding the hands of the dying, volunteering, working as an HIV/AIDS educator, putting my body on the line at ACT UP demonstrations, and going through it over and over again, on another level I probably I knew I was also gathering tools for my own survival. Sometimes resilience is absorbing huge setbacks—the loss of a close friend, a loved one—but most of the time it's just picking up the phone, calling a sick friend, making another doctor appointment, or taking another dose of meds.

Moreover, in Jackson's view the ability to refrain and resist addiction also demonstrates his resilience:

I give myself credit for not caving in to despair and turning to drugs or alcohol or obsessive unsafe sex, but that might be a matter of timing. I'd sampled drugs, alcohol, and reckless, anonymous sex in my high school and college years, long before my diagnosis, so my curiosity about that had long been satisfied, and fortunately I never felt intense emotional triggers around self-destructive behaviors.

As was examined in Chapter 5, new health challenges emerge for many of the men of the AIDS Generation. This includes ongoing concerns with anal cancer triggered by human papillomavirus (HPV) infection. Thus, with this in mind, Kerry also expressed his notions of resilience along the lines of health management but extended the ideas, like Richard, to address resilience in relation to the health complications of an aging HIV-infected body yet maintaining an attitude of hope and survival:

> To me it implies hope. For me it means that I know I will feel joy again in a way that is heightened by all the muck. It means getting stuck by needles every other month and still going to my doctor's appointments. It means checking for HPV every 6 months knowing full well there will be irregular cells and that the procedure will leave me incontinent for at least a month and just wearing the damn diapers anyway. It means having enough respect for those people who didn't have the option. It's about respect mingled with hope.

Ralph nested his understanding of resilience in terms of his history with AIDS, but not on his own health. Rather, he understood it in relation to the ongoing lives of the many who have survived and who continue to have fulfilling lives. In his view, managing and celebrating the disease is demonstrative of a resilient response, as opposed to letting the disease control one's life:

> Resilience is learned through examples, good and bad. Good being watching people grow and prosper and not let chronic illness take them down. Bad being the opposite and learning to choose positivity by seeing destruction in others who are unhappy, choosing to live lives of despair and sadness from what they may feel as being cheated by illness.

After our focus group in fall 2012, Kerry expressed a similar sentiment about being alive and celebrating life on his Facebook page:

> I was interviewed this summer for a book about long-term AIDS survivors and had the pleasure of meeting all the other interviewees last night. What a delightful group of men. While we all admitted to some fatigue, the room

was filled with hope and humor. It was one of the most "alive" rooms I have ever been in.

This notion of celebrating the collective resilience of the group also was expressed by Eddie:

> I think we are special. I think we are. And I think the testament to this is that we're all still here. And we all, regardless of whatever we've been through, seems like we're all still happy to be alive.

These ideas shared by the men of the AIDS Generation evoke a very grand and multifaceted conception of resilience. They understand their resilience in terms of not only their physical lives but also their emotions and their social engagement and cohesion. This idea of attending to the whole has permeated every aspect of this volume and is particularly relevant in the current state of the HIV epidemic. In recent times, efforts to address the ongoing epidemic in our country and, in fact, the world have been driven by biomedical advances. These include targeting, testing, and treating those who are infected and preventing infection with the use of HIV antivirals in the form of pre-exposure prophylaxis (PrEP; e.g., Grant et al., 2010). Although certainly significant, these biomedical approaches are advancing without a fully informed understanding of the multifaceted nature of the disease. HIV is a disease that is more than simply a virus, and failure to attend to the psychological and social aspects of this epidemic may limit the effectiveness of these biomedical advances, as recently noted in a resolution from the American Psychological Association (2012) that I helped to craft, which in part states:

> HIV/STI prevention research teams of the future must bridge biomedical and behavioral approaches and develop new combination approaches that consider biological, cognitive, attitudinal, affective, behavioral, gender, familial, developmental, cultural, educational, social, racial, linguistic, socioeconomic, religious, and environmental factors....

We barely understand how individuals will take and adhere to PrEP, and we clearly know that despite our best efforts, for every 100 Americans who are living with HIV, only 28 achieve full viral suppression through treatment (CDC, 2012e). The latter, known as the treatment cascade, reflects the idea that combatting HIV will require more than simply attending to the pathogen. Instead, we must attend to the whole person.

This holistic approach to disease management and ultimately to survival is the approach the men of the AIDS Generation espoused. Any health care provider who simply attends to the medical aspects of the disease and adheres to a biomedical model rather than a biopsychosocial one is providing a disservice to her or his patients, and to our war against this epidemic. The men of the AIDS Generation demonstrated their resilience by intelligently attending to the whole of their lives. And when this stops, all is lost. I was reminded of this again today, December 18, 2012, when ACT UP pioneer Spencer Cox died at age 44—another great loss for the AIDS Generation and for our society.

Demonstrations of Resilience

Throughout the course of this volume, the stories of the men of the AIDS Generation demonstrate resilience. It is evident in every utterance of these men and these quotes that I have shared with the reader. These demonstrations of resilience were evidenced even before they were diagnosed with AIDS, as young men and boys learning to negotiate their sexuality in a heteronormative and often homophobic and discriminatory world. It was evidenced in the manner in which they reacted to their diagnoses and the ongoing death around them. It is reflected in the strategies they used to survive and to attend to their physical, emotional, and social well-being. And it is evident in their lives today as they manage the process of aging.

It would be shortsighted and insincere of me to assert that all of the actions and behaviors of the AIDS Generation men were demonstrative of resilience. Some, like Bobby, avoided addressing their disease by immersing themselves in a world of substance use, that substance primarily being alcohol for Bobby. Others, like Tyronne, sold their HIV medications to pay for illicit drugs and a life of escape. And Richard and Andre engaged in unabashed sexual adventurism, perhaps as means of survival, but not necessarily a characteristic one would consider resilient. Yet even in these situations, there was an ultimate breakthrough that led to a life defined by more active than avoidant coping, as is demonstrated in the story of John. I digress to state one critical point—sex was one of the few pleasures for some of the men of the AIDS Generation, and "risky" sex is not simply and solely a function of mental illness as posited by some, including Murray and Adam (2001).

The extant literature has examined evidence for resilience that HIV-positive individuals bring to older adulthood. Siegel, Raveis, and Karus

(1998) reported that with age comes greater wisdom and increased respect for health and life. This is certainly noted in some of the stories of the men with whom I spoke. Particularly salient are the stories of Tyronne, Bobby, and Andre, who battled their substance use and denial of HIV as they emerged into their 40s and 50s. This too is the case for Eddie, who now at age 50 and after a complicated and often disjointed lifestyle has become an advocate, spokesman, and mentor for a new generation of young men living with the disease. In a 2005 study, Vance and Woodley noted that the resilience demonstrated by older HIV-positive adults emanates from their social support. This notion of social capital was very evident in the stories of almost all of the men with whom I spoke, who indicated such support from friends and family, as well as boyfriends, partners, and husbands. When such social capital was perceived as limited, as was the case for Kerry in relation to his work-related social network and his inability to identify a circle of men like himself, a sense of despair ensued. Moreover, although social support may be posited as a source of resilience for aging seropositive individuals, this condition was also evident throughout the course of many of the men's lives. Their engagement with activist organizations, their roles as spokesmen for HIV prevention and awareness, their care for those in their social circles who were dying while they lived, and their expression of the disease through their art all speak to the resilient nature of the men of the AIDS Generation.

Emlet et al. (2011, p. 1010) indicate, "Practitioners should identify and implement methods for assessing resilience among older HIV-infected individuals." I accept this notion but take it one step further. We must also understand the resilience of all those who are infected with HIV across their life spans as their resilience in early adulthood likely informs their resilience as older adults. That is to say that the men of the AIDS Generation do not simply present as resilient as they age; rather, their very nature was informed by resilience throughout the course of their lives as they battled to stay alive. This resilience, or competency, is in effect informed by having lived through the AIDS crisis (Emlet et al., 2011), an idea first brought to light when the advantages of living with and aging with HIV/AIDS were documented by Karolyn Siegel and her colleagues (1998). Despite the bumps in the road to middle age along the way, some of which were self-created, they each attended to their whole selves and forged ahead. Some adapted and demonstrated resilience earlier than others, as was the case of Christopher and Ryan, who immediately took proactive steps after their surprising diagnoses; of Patrick, who continued to attend to his body through his dance; of Jackson, as a member of ACT UP, who stood on the front lines demanding a cure for AIDS be found; and of Gianni, who simply refused to put his life on hold. What is common to all these men is that they all kept moving forward—the will to live, despite the grimmest prospects, is the most illustrative aspect of their resilient natures. It is this aspect of their being that directed them to self-care physically, psychologically, and socially. Perseverance and optimism underlie this will to live and forge ahead and is supported by the literature (Wagnild, 2009). Our brother, Spencer Cox, also had this will to live, until he didn't.

This will to live as the indicator of resilience may also be framed as a derivative of self-acceptance. The men of the AIDS Generation, at some point after their diagnoses, demonstrated this self-acceptance. For some it was immediate, whereas others delayed fully accepting their lives as HIV-positive gay men, diagnosed at a time of little hope. Regardless of where along the life continuum this occurred, each of the men did eventually reach a point where he integrated HIV into his life. This is not to say that the men defined their entire identities by their HIV. On the contrary, they embedded HIV into the contexts of their lives. My own experience has shown me that those in my life who fully defined their lives by their disease were the ones who also evidenced the greatest despair and stagnation. This is also supported by the work of Siegel and her colleagues (1998), who note that the latter prevents one from moving forward, and Emlet et al. (2011) indicate the beneficial effects of optimism. This optimistic approach has been evidenced throughout this volume and supported by how the men handled their diagnoses and the epidemic in their community, the strategies they enacted to remain viable, and the manner in which each is handling the process of aging.

The resilience of the men of the AIDS Generation is first demonstrated in the story of their diagnoses and their handling of this life-alerting event. This fortitude of spirit was evidenced despite the fact that many of the men were informed that their lives would end in 2 or so years after receiving the news (the "myth of two"). What proved to be a proactive response to the diagnosis followed a period of disconnection that I have described as "the pause" in Chapter 4. This disconnection was experienced physically and emotionally, as demonstrated in the stories of Gianni and Ralph, who quickly had to compose themselves because this news was delivered to them via telephone and while each was at his place of work. Tellingly, and after managing this period of disequilibrium, many of the men, including Kerry and Richard, then considered their "next steps"—what proactive approaches they would enact toward their diagnoses. This reaction is highly illustrative of resilience. This very dark moment was followed by a period of planning and forging ahead for almost all of the men with whom I spoke. For others, like Hal, the time for planning and action came after recovering from a life-threatening illness, which accompanied their diagnosis with AIDS. In the end, this power to move on and drive to live and triumph was ever-present in my conversations with the men of the AIDS Generation and was manifested among all of the men, whether the diagnosis was expected or unexpected and in the context of an epoch of the epidemic in which there were few indicators that one should have such hope of survival.

Also indicative of resilience is the manner in which the men of the AIDS Generation managed their own lives while facing the deaths of so many in their social circles including partners, lovers, and close friends. Antoine detailed the loss of all those he had met as a gay man and who had become his family of 40, only 3 of whom are alive today, and Ralph described how he continued to live his life while the devastation of the epidemic was decimating his community in San Francisco. For all of us, infected or not, the decade between 1985 and 1995 was characterized by endless deaths, memorial after memorial, and the loss of all those we loved. None of us were spared, and it would have been easy to retreat. But we did not and we triumphed. As a population, we continued to fight for our lives, for our rights, and in the memories of those we had lost. We knew a better day would have to come. This behavior is also illustrative of our individual and collective resilience. We would not give up, and in 1996 the epidemic took a turn. Still, we are not spared death from this epidemic, as I was recently reminded with the death of Spencer. I was inconsolable after receiving the news. His death reminded me how tired I was of fighting this disease—how tired we all are.

Perhaps the greatest evidence for the resilient nature of these men can be noted in the strategies they enacted to survive the epidemic. In Chapter 4, I examined the various approaches the men enacted to attend to their physical, emotional, and social well-being. This attendance to the whole self and to maintaining health in all aspects in one's life was a major undertaking for the men of the AIDS Generation. In a time of little hope, they sought solutions that they believed would maintain their viability. They enacted these strategies and were hopeful that their actions would reap beneficial outcomes and extend their lives. These approaches, like many of the efforts developed at the earliest AIDS service organizations (ASOs), were developed quickly and in response to the surge of the epidemic. There were no evidence-based interventions, there were no fool-proof treatments, and there was only a minimal understanding of how the disease would progress in each of their lives. All of these actions in light of dire circumstances demonstrate resilience—the tendency to keep moving forward in proactive and meaningful manners despite the shadow that AIDS was casting in each of their lives.

Tellingly, there was no lock-step pattern of actions the men of the AIDS Generation undertook to combat the virus. Each, to the best of his ability and to the best of his own knowledge, acted accordingly. Using what little information was available in the early days of AIDS and relying more often on instinct than knowledge, each fashioned an approach to life and to survival. In the first decade of AIDS this was often more art than science, and the strategies were directed by a survival instinct.

Most important and relevant to the notion of resilience is that the men of the AIDS Generation attended to the entirety of their existences (physical, emotional, and social). In the physical domain this included engaging in health-promoting behaviors such as exercise and the administration of supplements, eliminating potentially damaging behaviors such as substance use, and attending to the messages that the body provided to each man in close relationship with his health care team. Emotionally, the men of the AIDS Generation attempted to alleviate their lives of psychological burdens presented by the experiences of a lifetime of pain and loss through which they were living. They found comfort in their friends and loved ones, in the enactment of therapeutic processes whether individually or in groups, and through the loving partnerships they formed. Activism, engagement in support groups, and immersion with others with the same condition provided the social nurturing required by the men and enhanced their social capital. Ultimately, these strategies, indicative of resilience, allow the men to enhance and bolster their spirits to live and thrive beyond the immediate conditions created by their infections.

How the men of the AIDS Generation are aging with HIV is also illustrative of their resilience. In the last half of 2012, I came to know the men of the AIDS Generation very well. In our ongoing dialogues, either formally through the interview or focus group process or informally through our interactions online, what became apparent is that almost always their understanding of their lives today was characterized by hope and appreciation. Certainly, as was discussed in Chapter 5, the process of aging has created additional complications in the lives of these men—those of an aging body that takes longer to heal, those of a social condition in which older gay men are often invisible, and those of struggles with trying to make sense of one's place in the world and one's legacy. Yet despite these hurdles, the voice emanating from most of the men was one of hope and love of life. Their resilience is evidenced in the manner in which each is negotiating his memories of the past and of the loss experienced over the last three decades. Patrick described these feelings that were ignited in the summer of 2012 as he viewed the AIDS Memorial Quilt in Washington, DC. Bobby and John were reminded as they created their guest list for their wedding. Yet even as these events and others like them triggered great sadness, the men of the AIDS Generation demonstrated a fortitude in confronting the situations, reflecting on the past and what has transpired, and moving forward with their lives. These actions too are demonstrative of resilience.

I will admit that working on this volume has taken an emotional toll on me. I had neatly compartmentalized my emotions around this epidemic and the losses I have experienced. Through my work, I have come to intellectualize the AIDS epidemic and the havoc it has created in my life. Yet in writing, I could not escape the past, the loss of so many, and my own personal struggles, and for 1 month I was paralyzed in my attempts to write. It would have been easy to abandon the book because these emotions were so overwhelming. Yet giving up is also not part of my nature, and like the men of the AIDS Generation, I confronted my past head on and moved forward. I too needed to prove that I was resilient, that adversity would not stand in my way, and that I would forge ahead with this work and with my life. Like John, who described in Chapter 5 his need to rekindle his memories of the past to move on, I too needed to reimmerse myself in the depths of the despair I experienced to move ahead. Giving up was never an option for me, and defeat was never an option for the men of the AIDS Generation, a characteristic that is very much part of each of their constitutions as they now live through their middle age.

The resilience of these older men, these men of the AIDS Generation, is evident in our larger community. It seems that collectively we are all grappling with our legacies, making sense of our places in the world, and preparing for the later stages of life. This is likely true for all men in my generation, HIV-positive or HIV-negative, as we try to understand what we have experienced. My friend David France accomplished this through his beautiful documentary, Eddie through his mentoring of younger HIV-positive men, Kerry in his efforts to convene men like him to create a network, Ryan through his ongoing efforts with AIDS activist groups, Patrick through the sharing of his own life stories with his clients who are confronting their own health struggles, Richard through the performance of his musical around the world, John and Bobby through the melding of their lives as a married couple, and I through the writing of this book.

These acts of all of us, us older men, are very evident of a resilient nature. Despair will not characterize our lives even at this more advanced age. Rather, we will channel the losses and the pain and create a better existence for ourselves and for society at large. This is what it means to be resilient.

Sources of Resilience

The behavioral and psychological literature has attempted to delineate sources of resilience—how one develops a resilient approach to life. Wagnild (2003) posits that social supports in the form of families and communities foster resilience in individuals; others, like Rutter (1987), suggest it is a personal trait that is unique to each person. The question that continually is raised by social scientists is, "Is resilience best categorized as a process, an individual trait, a dynamic developmental process, an outcome, or all of the above?" (Zautra, Hall, & Murray, 2010, p. 4).

Although the sources of resilience are still debated in the literature, there is general agreement that resilience is a means of maintaining or regaining mental health in response to adversity or as a positive adaptation, as suggested by Herrman et al. (2011), or the ability to respond to and/or cope with stressful situations such as trauma, death, family conflict, or substance use (Masten & Powell, 2003; Resnick, 2000; Roosa, 2000), conditions that in the case of the men of the AIDS Generation are primarily but not entirely defined by the HIV epidemic.

Much of the research on resilience is derived from studies of childhood (e.g., Chapman et al., 2004), which indicate that for some children adverse life events such as emotional abuse may lead to psychopathology in adulthood, but that this is not the case for all. In effect, this finding suggests that resilience at any point in one's life is the result of the interaction of individual attributes and social context (Herrman et al., 2011), and that resilience is not a trait but rather a dynamic and interactive process of the person with his surroundings and his emotions and cognitions. Such an understanding of the interplay between person and environment in fostering resilience has also been evidenced in older adults (Rapp, 1998) and is known as a strength perspective (Emlet et al., 2011). Moreover, Herrman et al. (2011) suggest that resilience emanates from an interaction of personal, biological, and environmental-social factors and provide support from the literature for such a model.

This multifaceted consideration of resilience aligns with my own approach to understanding health and well-being, which is informed entirely by a biopsychosocial perspective (Engel, 1977). Just as HIV disease is not simply a biological condition, so too resilience cannot be understood solely as psychological phenomenon. A purely biomedical approach to HIV is insufficient, and a purely psychological interpretation of resilience is also lacking in this regard. That is all to say that it is no longer sufficient to consider resilience solely in the domain of developmental psychology (Luthar, 2006), and that we must consider the whole person as we examine resilient responses. During our conversations, Patrick shared a story about a woman he trains, which expressed this conception clearly, indicative of how the men of the AIDS Generation have cared for themselves:

> Another woman approached me and said it was my personal story that inspired her in her work as a medical professional. That she was so overwhelmed by sick people, she was losing sight of the fact that each person has a story, a history, friends and family who are all affected by how she dealt with each individual patient. That she could step back and see them as human beings and not just another problem to solve.

It is beyond the scope of this volume to fully examine the extant literature on resilience. Still, it is worth noting the most recent work of Zautra et al. (2010), who posit that individuals who are resilient are quick to reestablish physiological, psychological, and social equilibrium following stressful events. This was very much the case for many of the men of the AIDS Generation, such as Jackson, Kerry, Patrick, and Gianni, as they sought to establish their lives postdiagnosis. For others, who took longer to reestablish their lives, such as Eddie, Andre, and Bobby, one may argue that their reactions were less resilient, although I would argue that their ultimate confrontation of the disease demonstrated resilience, albeit at a slower pace. A second characteristic of resilience is sustainability, defined by Bonanno (2004) as the ability to continue forward in the face of adversity. In this regard all of the men with whom I spoke demonstrated resilience. None refused to continue living and each to the best of his ability moved his life forward, even when there was little hope for a future.

During the course of our conversations, I asked the men of the AIDS Generation to identify the sources of their resilience. What emerged predominantly in the men's understanding is the role that their parents and the environments in which they were raised played in developing their resilience. Patrick acknowledged the role his parents played as follows:

Thank you mom and dad for teaching me to not give up. If you want your dreams then be ready to commit to hard work. If things don't work out the way you planned then there is a reason so be ready to change your thinking.

This sentiment and idea were shared by Kerry, who said, "My parents taught me unconditional love and infused me with a wonderful sense of humor. None of this survival would be possible without either." And Jackson furthered this idea and expressed a thought that captures the role that both person and environment may play in developing resilience and provided a guide for his life:

Both my parents are from South Georgia. I come from healthy, farm stock and credit my mom and dad with instilling in me a shoulder-to-the-wheel Protestant work ethic and self-discipline. I'm thankful for the steadfast emotional support I've received from my entire family. I had both nature and nurture on my side, and they served as an important blueprint.

Finally, Christopher expressed his ideas as follows:

I'm not exactly sure where my own resilience comes from but my guess is that some of it is learned and some of it is innate. Looking back I definitely think my parents had a role in it. While neither of them ever dealt with a chronic or life-threatening illness, both have overcome a lot of adversity in their lives, my mom in particular. For me, birth order definitely played a role, being the—in the middle of two brothers, I got it from both sides and I've been forced to be flexible and adjust.

However, the men also described other life experiences that bolstered or informed their resilience. This was the case for Ralph, who grew up in large family in Utah and who acknowledges the important role of parents. But this was not his reality:

Some may learn by caring family and friends. Not me, my parents were assholes and others choose to learn from life experiences.

And for Patrick, his belief system helped him further develop his resilience: "Thank you Course in Miracles for teaching me that even the littlest change in perception is a true miracle. If I don't experience miracles often then something is wrong." And Jackson recognizes his own efforts: "But I've done a lot of work myself. I dedicate a lot of my life energy to preserving and protecting my health."

In listening to the men of the AIDS Generation and in reimmersing myself in their narratives on many occasions, what became clear to me is that for all of them, resilience developed in their childhoods as young men grappling with their sexuality. Most did not make this connection, other than Christopher, who said the following with regard to how he developed his resilience:

> I also think that wrestling with my own sexuality and trying to navigate through that in my teenage years taught me how to just "keep pushing" and to do what needed to be done.

That statement rings loudly and clearly and honestly. I know it is true for my own life experiences, and I see it clearly in the life experiences of all of the men with whom I spoke. Even if parents were loving and supportive, as was the case for John and Kerry (and for me), this did not ameliorate the burdens experienced being raised in a heteronormative and often discriminatory world in which men were portrayed as weak, effeminate, and sickly. I spoke to this issue more fully in Chapter 1.

The men of the AIDS Generation came of age in the 1970s and early 1980s, shortly after the Stonewall Riots and the beginning of the gay rights movement. In the some 40 years since that time, much progress has been made toward protecting the rights of LGBT individuals. It is likely that more progress would have been made if the AIDS epidemic had not derailed us and fueled the venom and hatred of many in our society toward sexual minority individuals, even my own city's mayor in the 1980s, whose own internalized homophobia kept him in the closet for his entire life. This is all to say that for many of us, the process of coming out was fraught with questions and complications. Few if any role models existed. And being gay was still taboo and anathema in the eyes of many. None of us knew that our blue-collar fathers ultimately could and would be loving and accepting. We didn't know. There were no television programs like *Glee*, depicting Kurt Hummel and the love and acceptance and support of his auto-mechanic father; we did not live in a society where the majority of the population supports marriage equality and where we could have married the man we loved; openly gay and proud celebrities like Neil Patrick Harris and Anderson Cooper were not part of our existence in these formative years. In the absence of these conditions, all of us, as children and adolescents, lived our lives secretly and quietly in hopes that one day we could live our lives fully and openly.

It is this negotiation and this struggle that I firmly believe formed our individual and collective constitutions and fostered the resilience evident in so many of the men of the AIDS Generation. In fact, after living through this struggle and experiencing both overt and silent stigma and victimization, HIV was in some ways just another burden with which we had to contend. And we had a lifetime of learning how to manage burdens. One learns how to be resilient if one has spent years suppressing and hiding who one really is.

As young boys with our sexuality emerging, many of us needed to develop strategies for survival. This is not to say that we were confronting a deadly virus. Rather, we needed to maintain our emotional lives while managing the fear of being different, as shown in Bobby's story as a young man in New Orleans; we were required to navigate our social contexts in schools and playgrounds and family events with caution, hiding our true identities, as evidenced in Ralph's life story growing up in Utah; and many of us had to attend to our bodies, building our strength and power in defense of our lives from those bullies who took pleasure in harassing us, as was the case for John while he was growing up on the east end of Long Island. We as young gay men had no choice but to manage all of this while attempting to maintain a sense of integrity in our lives and managing the demands that life was placing upon us. Is there any question why so many turned to substance use as young men? How could one not try to escape the conditions of life after years of living with burdens and secrets and fears of being "caught"?

John Genke (2004), a social worker who has worked with many gay men, posits that negotiating the coming-out process provides gay men with an advantage over their straight counterparts, in part due to the stigma and loss that gay men must confront at much younger ages. This conception is also supported by the work of my colleague Anthony D'Augelli (1994), who suggests that the experience of coming out and its associated crises provide gay men with the ability to understand all future life crises. I would further suggest that it provides gay men with the resilience to handle such future life crises, as evidenced in the actions and strategies of the men of the AIDS Generation.

In such conditions, how could we also not learn how to be resilient, a quality that helped us to survive HIV? Our situations as young boys required that we be creative and clever and think outside the box. Our resilience emerged in us naturally as we navigated our childhoods and teenage years trying to make sense of our places in the world, fearing who we were, and managing to remain intact. Perhaps it was our struggles with our sexual orientation that provided us with the fortitude and savvy to combat the AIDS epidemic. In this regard and in consideration of the aging process for gay men, Genke (2004, p. 82) further asserts, "This [the life crises of coming out] may account for some of the resiliency…" noted in aging gay men. Moreover, this resilience continued to developed in the lives of these young men even after the coming-out process as they emerged into their adulthood and confronted the demands for physical perfection in the gay community, the challenge of learning how to negotiate a relationship with another man in the absence of any role modeling, the struggle to develop and understand one's self-worth, the unexpected storm of AIDS and the ensuing losses, and, for many of the men of the AIDS Generation, the challenge of substance use and the complications of trying to reconcile a life as a veteran of the AIDS epidemic. All of these conditions have been described in the preceding chapters as they manifested in the lives of the men with whom I spoke. It is safe to say that the resilience of the men of the AIDS Generation was born in their childhoods but was also strengthened through a life full of struggles, where ultimately HIV emerged as yet another burden. Gianni captured this idea perfectly when he said:

> Seriously, I was gay, and I had to hide it all my life until I was on my own, until I left home and this is 1981. I did the whole straight thing in high school to get by because that's what I thought I needed to do. And I passed. Then days into being—having sex with a man, AIDS is all around. Come on, seriously. And that guy ends up dying a few years later. And it's just been one thing after another ever since.

Thus, the story of HIV and the men of the AIDS Generation is the story of the lives of a generation of gay men who emerged into their adulthood at a most inopportune time, but who managed through their determination and knowledge from a lifetime of challenges to reach middle age. Their diagnoses with HIV may be a point of inflection in their lives, but their resilience before and after the diagnosis is the true story of their lives.

Sharing Strategies for Resilience

Recently I had the opportunity to meet Thomas, a remarkable young man in his 20s who is a student at NYU. An accomplished musician, he is also a gay man living with HIV. My immediate reaction was to take this man under my wing and to protect him. I introduced him to Richard, the musician you have come to know in this volume, with whom he formed an immediate bond. As I think about this young man, I am reminded of another ability of our generation that often goes untapped—that of acting as mentors to a new generation of young gay men also confronting this disease that continues to affect our population. Eddie perfectly understands this role and enacts it with great pride. This, however, remains an untapped opportunity for many of us—those of us who have confronted the disease for decades working with those who are only beginning their journeys. I raise this issue because I believe that what we have learned over the years and how we have demonstrated our resilience as a generation of men can only help to enhance the life of Thomas and all of these younger men who too are affected by this epidemic.

In Chapter 5, I examined the reactions of the men of the AIDS Generation to the rising number of infections in those under age 30. During our conversations, many of those with whom I spoke expressed dismay and to some extent anger at the current situation, suggesting that these young men "should know better." This reaction is summarized in the words of Bobby, which takes these reactions a step further by connecting the success and survival of long-term survivors, like himself, to the rising infection rates:

> I can picture how some younger men may simply not care if they're infected with HIV because they see men like us who are long-term survivors and they think, "I can deal with this. The precautions aren't worth the trouble."
> I wish they knew us personally, and could hear the endless litany of injections, infections, pills, regimens, routines...the everyday indignations of diarrhea, fatigue, worry...the emotional toll on ourselves and our families.

Jackson also expressed a similar sentiment toward these newly infected young gay men:

> I feel a combination of sympathy, frustration, helplessness, and rage. I want to shake them, hold them, comfort them, and protect them.

During our conversations, many of the men of the AIDS Generation came to understand the challenges that these young gay men experience coming out, shaping their identities, and forming their lives. I directed all of them to an article I had written titled "Discrimination and Homophobia Fuel the

HIV Epidemic in Gay and Bisexual Men" (Halkitis, 2012a) and expressed my own belief that social policies in the United States such as the Defense of Marriage Act continue to undermine the well-being of our population (Halkitis, 2012b). Although I am not certain all were completely convinced of my proposition, I believe that I was able to help move the conversation from one of blame to one of greater compassion for these young men. If we, the men of the AIDS Generation, were blindsided by the AIDS epidemic, then perhaps our greatest responsibility is to ensure that a new generation of men are better equipped intellectually and emotionally to combat this disease—perhaps there is knowledge in our own experiences that can serve as learning opportunities for those newly infected and those at risk. Perhaps it is time for us to take our place as the elder statesmen of this population and provide these young men with the guidance that can be bestowed from our years of experience. Having survived the epidemic and despite our battle scars and fatigue, the men of the AIDS Generation are obligated to embrace such a role. How our resilience informed many of our lives can perhaps serve as a model for those who at a very young age are also grappling with this disease.

To this point, I directly asked the men of the AIDS Generation what advice they would give to a young gay man newly infected with HIV. Richard described it as follows:

> I think they can learn that with great challenges comes great rewards. The personal pride that I feel from having fought so hard and endured so much has made my life rich with the feeling of accomplishment. Not just for people with HIV, but so many friends and followers have told me that by watching me fight and survive, it gives them the strength to do the same. And it happens so often that I almost begin to take it for granted.
>
> I remember one young man who was suffering from depression. He felt like he could not go on. But when he found my blog and read my story, he wrote to me, "I thought if he can get through what he's gotten through, then I know things will come out better if I also survive." At the pit of his despair, it seemed to him that darkness was the only thing possible. That this is what the world is. But by being open with my struggle, he saw that there is light. He just needs to get through the blackness to find that light.

In many of the responses, there was a sense of empowerment. Many of the men were speaking to their resilience, although they did not necessarily use that word, and their reactions were informative of how they have managed their disease (which is illustrative of resilience) and how these experiences could be imparted to help others. Patrick made meaning of this sharing of knowledge and experiences as follows:

> To those who find themselves new to the HIV world I would say that even though it sounds awful, this is a gift, a lesson, embrace it and learn everything you can about the disease. Knowledge is power and strength too. Adapt, adjust your course, be flexible and ready to change your mind about things...often.

Similarly, John delineates the challenges he faced, the challenges he continues to face, and how he confronts these elements of his life as a cautionary lesson to all who might be at risk for HIV or anyone newly infected when he presents at local area high schools:

> I'm alive today due to a combination of things; the angels and miracles that conspired to get me sober, staying sober, a positive mental attitude once I got off the pity pot and got sober, a higher power, good genes, my family and friends, and the miracles of modern medicine. I developed full-blown AIDS in 1997 when my T cells dropped below 200, I had KS as well as cryptococcal meningitis, but fortunately for me the new HIV cocktail arrived and changed everything for me. My T cells went up and all my AIDS-related diseases disappeared. But, as I tell students, there are three things you must remember about these new HIV drugs: they are very toxic, they stop working when the body develops resistance, and they are very expensive. So toxic that the only time I have ever been hospitalized was for two allergic reactions to HIV medication so severe that I nearly died....Last year, 2012, with the addition of Egrifta to my HIV regimen, my insurance company spent $55,000 on my HIV medications alone....Knowledge is power and my hope is that I give these students, gay and straight, the knowledge to make sound decisions in the future and maybe, if I am truly as blessed as I believe I am, one of them will live long enough to discover the cure to this disease.

For Kerry, the lesson he imparts is one of self-love, and more importantly of coming together as a community, an idea upon which he reflected many times during our conversations:

> I always think of it as a cautionary tale. A warning to slow it down. A call to love one another as a community. A call to love yourself and for the newly infected an inspiration to stay alive just like us.

This need for social support and love was also evidenced in Jackson's recommendation:

> I would encourage younger HIV positives to seek out people who are not only supportive and nurturing but also people who aren't afraid to call us on our bullshit. It's important for all of us—young, old, positive, and negative—to surround ourselves with people who will love us, be honest with us, and urge us to be our best selves. And we need to love those people back the same way. Because ultimately, what will survive of all of us is love.

These notions of love for others, self-love and acceptance, sorting through one's life, and adjusting and accommodating are also evident in the advice provided by Bobby:

> If I met someone newly infected, I would encourage him to go to the mountaintop, emotionally speaking. Spend some time sorting through the range of emotions he'll encounter, which would certainly include anger at himself and whoever infected him, shame, doubt, fear. I'd want him to consider the hard question: "What do I deserve in my life?" I didn't consider that hard question until it was too late. My core beliefs about myself pre-HIV and for a considerable amount of time after exposure seem, in retrospect, to lead inexorably to my infection. I was damaged goods and "deserved" bad things. I took my sweet damn time finally addressing this deficit in myself, and now believe that I truly deserve health, life, love, friendship, career, community. Therefore, the decisions I make for myself reflect my growing self-love.

And for Christopher, the lessons of living with HIV that he has learned speak to not only those newly infected but also those living with other chronic conditions:

> I think people can see/learn that they can live very productive lives with HIV or another chronic illness. They can see that there are people out there that have been on the front lines fighting HIV and have lived to tell about it. I think Michael J. Fox said it best in his book *Always Looking Up*. I think this is true with my experience living with HIV/AIDS and would guess others have experienced it too. We've all been very resilient, because despite our setbacks, despite our really bad days... we've had a lot of those... we've all managed to look on the bright side of most situations and most important we've kept going.

To this point, what Michael J. Fox writes (2009, p. 6)

> For everything this disease has taken, something of greater value has been given...sometimes a marker that points me in a new direction I might not otherwise have traveled. So sure, it may be one step forward and two steps back, but after a time with Parkinson's, I've learned that what's important is making that one step count; always looking up.

Fox's voice is also indicative of a man with high levels of resilience. In the end, Jackson provides an all-encompassing understanding of how he has survived AIDS and how his experiences speak to anyone facing a chronic condition, acknowledging his advantages but also speaking to practical approaches all can espouse:

> I've had a lot of advantages that many people don't have—access to quality medical care, a strong support system of friends, family, and community, living in New York when AIDS, HIV was part of the conversation. And I was surrounded with role models, people who worked much harder than me, who were stronger, smarter, and more heroic who did not survive. So before I offer any advice I want to honor them and the lessons they taught me. I fully believe in the "grandmother cure"—eating right, getting exercise, and moderation. There are many reasons to be hopeful about facing HIV or any disease. Support and the tools for survival are available, sometimes in unexpected places. But you have to seek them out. That means doing the work, weeding through a lot of nonsense, and realizing that some strategies that work for other people won't work for you. But you won't find the support or the survival tools you need unless you fully embrace the world and its challenges....Everything I learned, I learned from musicals. This is an excerpt from a final scene in *Oklahoma*, when Aunt Eller teaches Laurey about resilience....The lesson is universal. It applies in the context of HIV/AIDS or any life-threatening illness.

To the reader who may not be familiar with the dialogue from *Oklahoma* (Rodgers & Hammerstein, 1942), it is shown below:

LAUREY: I don't see why this had to happen when everything was so fine.

AUNT ELLER: Now don't let your mind run on it.

LAUREY: [sobbing] I won't ever forget, I tell ya. Never will.

AUNT ELLER: That's alright, Laurey baby. You can't forget, just don't try to. Oh, lots of things happen to folks. Sickness, or bein' poor and hungry, bein' old and a feared to die. That's the way it is, cradle to grave. You can stand it. But there's just one way—you gotta be hardy. You gotta be! You can't deserve the sweet and tender in life unless'n you're tough!

The Workings of Resilience

As I conclude this book, I consider what the life stories of the men of the AIDS Generation have taught us about managing a disease once considered to always be life-threatening and now more often viewed as a chronic disease. This is by no means intended to be a theoretical paradigm; rather, my intention is to provide practical suggestions for those newly diagnosed with HIV and those in the health profession who work with their patients. These are the lessons I have derived from this journey I have taken with the men of the AIDS Generation. These guidelines are provided in clear and concise list format insomuch as they can function as a resource for those working with HIV-positive individuals or, perhaps, anyone living with a chronic and potentially life-threatening disease. Although I state these recommendations with regard to HIV, I believe that they are transferable to those facing similarly demanding health conditions. Fearing these might be interpreted as a whimsical, trite, self-help guide as put forward by some of my colleagues in search of fame and glory, I do not elaborate on these recommendations. Instead, I leave these open to interpretation as guideposts that can be interested by each as he or she best sees fit:

1. Confront and accept HIV, and do not define your life solely by HIV.
2. Attend to all aspects of your health, including the physical, emotional, and social aspects of your life.
3. Keep moving forward with all aspects of your life, and maintain a conscious will to live, thrive, and triumph.
4. Recognize that you are not alone in your battle against HIV, and build your networks of those who will fully embrace your life.
5. Enjoy all aspects of your life without fear of judgment from external forces, who may, in their judgment, fail to understand that the pleasures of life are still central.
6. Learn as much as you can about HIV and stay informed of the latest developments.

7. Develop a partnership with your HIV and other health care providers.

8. There is no one correct path to handling and addressing HIV; forge the path that works best for you.

9. Share your journey confronting HIV with those who are beginning theirs.

10. Recognize that there will be challenges with your health, but do not direct your life fearing these challenges before they emerge.

All of these strategies were very much enacted by the men of the AIDS Generation. Moreover, they are indicative of the will to survive shown by so many gay men in the early days of AIDS who struggled with the many unknowns of the disease but who attempted to make sense and garner some control over their lives (Weitz, 1989).

Final Thought

In January 2013, and as has been the case since 2005, I led an annual pilgrimage to London with graduate students to teach a course on HIV prevention and counseling—cross-cultural comparisons of responses to the epidemic. (London has always felt like home since my first trip here as a very young man and has been an inspirational environment for me.) As in years past, my colleague Angela Byrne, a highly respected clinical psychologist, presents on her work with HIV-positive individuals. Her lecture is always powerful as she shares case studies of some of those whom she has treated. Angela is soft-spoken and kind and every time I see her I am reminded of what an amazing therapist she must truly be.

This year, and prompted by my work on this volume, Angela presented a case study of a gay man named Ian. Ian, she said, is likely a member of "the AIDS Generation U.K." Ian's life story very much resembled the life experiences of the men of the AIDS Generation. At 48 years old, he too was experiencing the challenges of middle age and a negotiation of his life with HIV. And like many, Ian experienced an existential crisis of identity and legacy. For him, this condition led him to abandon his lifetime hobby of creating music and to move from his home in Earl's Court, which for men of my generation was a key center of gay life in the 1980s.

As Angela shared this story it became clear to me that Ian, like the men you have come to know in this book, was grappling and struggling with how to make sense of his life, especially now as he approached these more advanced years—after a lifetime of expecting never to reach this age.

Yet also like the men in this book, Ian confronted this struggle in a manner similar to which he confronted every challenge in his life living with HIV, including the multiple losses and devastation that he witnessed as a young man at the onset of the epidemic. He too demonstrated a resilience during the course of his life—a fortitude upon which he relied to manage this newest challenge brought forth by entering middle age. (Ian moved back to Earl's Court and began making mixing tapes as a reentry point to his music and after a short course of therapy with Angela.)

The story of Ian reminded me once again of the remarkable nature of my generation of gay men, of how we have managed our lives with dignity and respect and how our legacy is in fact the manner in which we lived our lives under the most hideous and horrifying of circumstances. These actions must be remembered and celebrated and should serve as a model for future generations of gay men, who I can only hope will live their lives under less cruel and perilous conditions.

While I was in London, I received a text message from my friend Kelly. The Oscar nominations had just been announced, and *How to Survive a Plague* had been nominated for Best Documentary. I read the text and smiled, realizing that our lives, the lives of the men of the AIDS Generation, were finally receiving the honor and respect that they deserved. In 2012, the pop singer Kelly Clarkson exclaimed, "What doesn't kill you makes you stronger." We, the men of the AIDS Generation, are strong; we are stronger having survived this plague. I stand in awe of the individual and collective resilience and triumphant spirits of these men, and I hope that this book effectively celebrates the stories of the men of the AIDS Generation, one of which is my own.

REFERENCES

Adhiyaman, V., Adhiyaman, S., & Sundaram, R. (2007). The Lazarus phenomenon. *Journal of the Royal Society of Medicine, 100*(12), 552–557. doi:10.1258/jrsm.100.12.552

AIDSinfo. (2012, September 13). An overview of Epivir (3TC, lamivudine). *The Body.* Retrieved from http://www.thebody.com/content/art4298.html

Altman, L. K. (1981, July 3). Rare cancer seen in 41 homosexuals. *The New York Times, 3.* Retrieved from http://www.nytimes.com/1981/07/03/us/rare-cancer-seen-in-41-homosexuals.html

Altman, L. K. (1982a, May 11). New homosexual disorder worries health officials. *The New York Times.* Retrieved from http://www.nytimes.com/1982/05/11/science/new-homosexual-disorder-worries-health-officials.html?pagewanted=all

Altman, L. K. (1982b, June 18). Clue found on homosexuals' precancer syndrome. *The New York Times.* Retrieved from http://www.nytimes.com/1982/06/18/us/clue-found-on-homosexuals-precancer-syndrome.html

American Psychological Association. (2012, February 25). *Combination biomedical and behavioral approaches to optimize HIV prevention.* Retrieved from http://www.apa.org/about/policy/biomedical-hiv.pdf

The Antiretroviral Therapy Cohort Collaboration. (2008). Life expectancy of individuals on combination antiretroviral therapy in high-income countries: A collaborative analysis of 14 cohort studies. *The Lancet, 372*(9635), 293–299.

Arias, E. (2011). United States life tables, 2007. *National Vital Statistics Reports, 59*(9), 1–60.

Armstrong, W. (2010, September). St. Vincent's remembers. *OUT, 197,* pp. 90–96, 148.

Appay, V., & Sauce, D. (2007). Immune activation and inflammation in HIV-1 infection: Causes and consequences. *Journal of Pathology, 214*(2), 231–241. doi:10.1002/path.2276

Appleby, P. R., Miller, L. C., & Rothspan, S. (1999). The paradox of trust for male couples: When risking is a part of loving. *Personal Relationships, 6*(1), 81–93. doi:10.1111/j.1475-6811.1999.tb00212.x

Aschengrau, A., & Seage, G. (2008). *Essentials of epidemiology in public health.* Sudbury, MA: Jones & Bartlett Learning.

Barré-Sinoussi, F., Chermann, J. C., Rey, F., Nugeyre, M. T., Chamaret, S., Gruest, J.,...Montagnier, L. (1983). Isolation of a T-lymphotropic retrovirus from a patient at risk for acquired immune deficiency syndrome (AIDS). *Science, 220*(4599), 868–871. doi:10.1126/science.6189183

Barroso, J. (1996). Focusing on living: Attitudinal approaches of long-term survivors of AIDS. *Issues in Mental health Nursing, 17*(5), 395–407. doi:10.3109/01612849609009409

Barroso, J. (1997). Reconstructing my life: Becoming a long-term survivor of AIDS. *Qualitative Health Research, 7*(1), 57–74. doi:10.1177/104973239700700104

Barroso, J., Buchanan, D., Tomlinson, P., & Van Servellen, G. (1997). Social support and long-term survivors of AIDS. *Western Journal of Nursing Research, 19*(5), 554–582. doi:10.1177/019394599701900502

Bayer, R. (1987). *Homosexuality and American psychiatry: The politics of diagnosis.* Princeton, NJ: Princeton University Press.

Bayer, R., Levine, C., & Wolf, S. M. (1986). HIV antibody screening, an ethical framework for evaluating proposed program. *Journal of the American Medical Association, 256*(13), 1768–1774. doi:10.1001/jama.256.13.1768

Bayer, R., & Oppenheimer, G. M. (2000). *AIDS doctors: Voices from the epidemic.* New York, NY: Oxford University Press.

Berger, J. (1985, October 3). Rock Hudson, screen idol, dies at 59. *The New York Times.* Retrieved from http://www.nytimes.com/1985/10/03/arts/rock-hudson-screen-idol-dies-at-59.html

Bernstein, J. (2012a, March 30). Not waiting to say goodbye. *The New York Times.* Retrieved from http://www.nytimes.com/2012/04/01/fashion/the-life-and-death-of-the-therapist-bob-bergeron.html?pagewanted=all

Bernstein, J. (2012b, December 12). A story of AIDS, from the beginning. *The New York Times.* Retrieved from http://www.nytimes.com/2012/12/13/fashion/how-to-survive-a-plague-provides-a-silver-lining-on-aids.html?pagewanted=1&_r=0&adxnnl=1&adxnnlx=1355411516-ZHuIoPSMWHSsAsLFXF%20bvw

Bernstein, J. (2013, February 22). Surviving AIDS but not the life that followed. *The New York Times.* Retrieved from http://www.nytimes.com/2013/02/24/fashion/what-really-killed-spencer-cox-aids-activist.html?pagewanted=all

Boissé, L., Gill, M. J., & Power, C. (2008). HIV infection of the central nervous system: Clinical features and neuropathogenesis. *Neurologic Clinics, 26*(3), 799–819. doi:10.1016/j.ncl.2008.04.002

Bonanno, G. A. (2004). Loss, trauma, and human resilience: Have we underestimated the human capacity to thrive after extremely aversive events? *American Psychologist, 59*(1), 20–28. doi:10.1037/0003-066X.59.1.20

Bower, J. E., Kemeny, M. E., Taylor, S. E., & Fahey, J. L. (1998). Cognitive processing, discovery of meaning, CD4 decline, and AIDS-related mortality among bereaved HIV-seropositive men. *Journal of Consulting and Clinical Psychology, 66*(6), 979. doi:10.1037/0022-006X.66.6.979

Bozzette, S. (2011). HIV and cardiovascular disease. *Clinical Infectious Diseases, 53*(1), 92–93. doi:10.1093/cid/cir275

Brand, M., & Markowitsch, H. J. (2010). Aging and decision-making: A neurocognitive perspective. *Gerontology, 56*(3), 319–324. doi:10.1159/000248829

Brennan-Ing, M., & Tax, A. (2013, March). *Forging a policy initiative on HIV & aging: Current directions and next steps.* Workshop presented at the Aging in America Conference, American Society on Aging, Chicago, IL.

Brookmeyer, R., Gail, M. H., & Polk, F. (1987). The prevalent cohort study and the acquired immunodeficiency syndrome. *American Journal of Epidemiology, 126*(1), 14–24.

Cahill, S., & Valadéz, R. (2012, June 29). Community-based approaches to HIV prevention that address antigay stigma. Retrieved from http://gmhc-online.blogspot.com/2012/06/community-based-approaches-to-hiv.html

Cahill, S., & Valadéz, R. (2013). Growing older with HIV/AIDS: New public health challenges. *American Journal of Public Health, 103*(3), e7–e15.

Callen, M. (1990). *Surviving AIDS.* New York, NY: HarperCollins.

Carr, A. (2000). HIV protease inhibitor-related lipodystrophy syndrome. *Clinical Infectious Diseases, 30*(2), 135–142.

Carr, A. (2003). HIV lipodystrophy: Risk factors, pathogenesis, diagnosis, and management. *AIDS, 17*, S141–S148.

Carr, A., & Cooper, D. A. (2000). Adverse effects of antiretroviral therapy. *The Lancet, 356*(9230), 1423–1430.

Catalan, J. (1999). Psychological problems in people with HIV infection. In J. Catalan (Ed.), *Mental health and HIV infection* (pp. 21–35). New York, NY: Routledge.

Cené, C. W., Akers, A. Y., Lloyd, S. W., Albritton, T., Powell Hammond, W., & Corbie-Smith, G. (2011). Understanding social capital and HIV risk in rural African American communities. *Journal of General Internal Medicine, 26*(7), 737–744. doi:10.1007/s11606-011-1646-4

Centers for Disease Control and Prevention. (1992). 1993 Revised classification system for HIV infection and expanded surveillance case definition for AIDS among adolescents and adults. *Morbidity and Morality Weekly Report Recommendation and Reports, 41*(RR-17), 1–19.

Centers for Disease Control and Prevention. (2001). HIV and AIDS—United States, 1981-2000. *Morbidity and Morality Weekly Report Recommendations and Reports, 50*(21), 430–434.

Centers for Disease Control and Prevention. (2010) *Establishing a holistic framework to reduce inequities in HIV, viral hepatitis, STDs, and tuberculosis in the United States.* Atlanta, GA: U.S. Department of Health and Human Services, Centers for Disease Control and Prevention.

Center for Disease Control and Prevention. (2012a). *AIDS trends.* Retrieved from http://www.cdc.gov/hiv/topics/surveillance/resources/slides/trends/index.htm

Centers for Disease Control & Prevention. (2012b, February). *HIV in the United States: At a glance.* Retrieved from http://www.cdc.gov/hiv/resources/factsheets/PDF/stats_basics_factsheet.pdf

Centers for Disease Control & Prevention. (2012c). HIV infections attributed to male-to-male sexual contact — Metropolitan statistical areas, United States and Puerto Rico, 2010. *Morbidity and Mortality Weekly Report, 61*(47), 962–966.

Centers for Disease Control and Prevention. (2012d, May). *HIV among gay and bisexual men.* Retrieved from http://www.cdc.gov/hiv/topics/msm/pdf/msm.pdf

Centers for Disease Control and Prevention. (2012e). *HIV in the United States: The stages of care.* Retrieved from http://www.cdc.gov/nchhstp/newsroom/docs/2012/Stages-of-CareFactSheet-508.pdf

Centers for Disease Control and Prevention. (2013a, February). *HIV surveillance report, 2011* (Vol. 23). Retrieved from http://www.cdc.gov/hiv/surveillance/resources/reports/2011report/pdf/2011_HIV_Surveillance_Report_vol_23.pdf

Centers for Disease Control & Prevention. (2013b). Diagnoses of HIV infection among adults aged 50 years and older in the United States and dependent areas, 2007–2010. *HIV Surveillance Supplemental Report, 18*(3), 1–70.

Chandra, A., Mosher, W. D., Copen, C., & Sionean, C. (2011). *Sexual behavior, sexual attraction, and sexual identity in the United States: Data from the 2006–2008 National Survey of Family Growth.* Atlanta, GA: U.S. Department of Health and Human Services, Centers for Disease Control and Prevention.

Chapman, D. P., Whitfiled, C. L., Felitti, V. J., Dube, S. R., Edwards, V. J., & Anda, R. F. (2004). Adverse childhood experiences and the risk of depressive disorders in childhood. *Journal of Affective Disorders, 82*(2), 217–225. doi:10.1016/j.jad.2003.12.013

Chochinov, H. M., Hack, T., Hassard, T., Kristijanson, L. J., McClement, S., & Harlos, M. (2005). Dignity therapy: A novel psychotherapeutic intervention for patients near the end of life. *Journal of Clinical Oncology, 23*(24), 5520–5525. doi:10.1200/JCO.2005.08.391

CNN. (2012, August 1). *Greg Louganis on HIV and Chick-Fil-A* [Video file]. Retrieved from http://www.youtube.com/watch?v=WNq6Bv6dOhI

Committee on Lesbian, Gay, Bisexual, and Transgender Health Issues and Research Gaps and Opportunities, Institute of Medicine. (2011). *The health of lesbian, gay, bisexual, and transgender people: Building a foundation for better understanding.* Washington, DC: National Academy Press.

Connor, S., & Kingman, S. (1988). *The search for the virus, the scientific discovery of AIDS and the quest for a cure.* New York, NY: Penguin Books.

Considine, A. (2011, December 31). Gay marriage victory still shadowed by AIDS. *The New York Times.* Retrieved from http://www.nytimes.com/2012/01/01/fashion/aids-casts-a-shadow-over-gay-marriage-victory.html?pagewanted=all&_r=0

Cook, P. F., Sousa, K. H., Matthews, E. E., Meek, P. M., & Kwong, J. (2011). Patterns of change in symptom clusters with HIV disease progression. *Journal of Pain Symptom Management, 42*(1), 12–23. doi:10.1016/j.jpainsymman.2010.09.021

Cotter, A. G., & Mallon, P. W. (2011). HIV infection and bone disease: Implications for an aging population. *Sexual Health, 8*(4), 493–501. doi:10.1071/SH11014#sthash.IyRP9w4b.dpuf

Cotter, A. G., & Powderly, W. G. (2011). Endocrine complications of human immunodeficiency virus infection: Hypogonadism, bone disease and tenofovir-related toxicity. *Best Practice & Research Clinical Endocrinology & Metabolism, 25*(3), 501–515. doi:10.1016/j.beem.2010.11.003

Crossley, M. L. (1999). Making sense of HIV infection: Discourse and adaptation to life with a long-term HIV positive diagnosis. *Health, 3*(1), 95–120. doi:10.1177/136345939900300104

Crothers, K., Huang, L., Goulet, J. L., Goetz, M. B., Bown, S. T., Rodriguez-Barradas, M. C.,...Justice, A. C. (2011). HIV infection and risk for incident pulmonary diseases in the combination antiretroviral therapy era. *American Journal of Respiratory and Critical Care Medicine, 183*(3), 388–395. doi:10.1164/rccm.201006-0836OC

Crum, N. F., Spencer, C. R., & Amling, C. L. (2004). Prostate carcinoma among men with human immunodeficiency virus infection. *Cancer, 101*(2), 294–299. doi:10.1002/cncr.20389

D'Augelli, A. R. (1994). Lesbian and gay male development: Steps toward an analysis of lesbians' and gay men's lives. In B. Greene & G. Herek (Eds.), *Psychological perspectives on lesbian and gay issues, Vol. 1: Lesbian & gay psychology: Theory, research and clinical applications* (pp. 118–132). Thousand Oaks, CA: Sage.

Davies, M. L. (1997). Shattered assumptions: Time and the experience of long-term HIV-positivity. *Social Science & Medicine, 44*(5), 561–571. doi:10.1016/S0277-9536(96)00177-3

Department of Health and Human Services. (2005, October). Side effects of anti-HIV medications. *Health Information for Patients.* Retrieved from http://aidsinfo.nih.gov/ContentFiles/SideEffectAnitHIVMeds_cbrochure_en.pdf

Dewar, R., Goldstein, D., & Maldarelli, F. (2009). Diagnosis of human immunodeficiency virus infection. In G. L. Mandell, G. E. Bennett, & R. Dolins (Eds.), *Principles and practice of infectious diseases* (7th ed., pp. 1663–1686). Philadelphia, PA: Elsevier Churchill Livingstone.

Doka, K. J. (2009). *Counseling individuals with life-threatening illness.* New York, NY: Springer Publishing Company.

Doty, M. (1995). Is there a future? In M. Howe & M. Klein (Eds.), *In the company of my solitude: American writing from the AIDS pandemic* (pp. 3–12). New York, NY: Persea Books.

Duberman, M. B. (1994). *Stonewall.* New York, NY: Plume.

Dubrow, R., Silverberg, M. J., Park, L. S., Crothers, K., & Justice, A. C. (2012). HIV infection, aging, and immune function: Implications for cancer risk and prevention. *Current Opinion in Oncology, 24*(5), 506–516. doi:10.1097/CCO.0b013e328355e131

Eaton, L. A., West, T. V., Kenny, D. A., & Kalichman, S. C. (2009). HIV transmission risk among HIV seroconcordant and serodiscordant couples: Dyadic processes of partner selection. *AIDS and Behavior, 13*(2), 185–195. doi:10.1007/s10461-008-9480-3

Emlet, C. A., Tozay, S., & Raveis, V. H. (2011). "I'm not going to die from the AIDS": resilience in aging with HIV disease. *The Gerontologist, 51*(1), 101–111. doi:10.1093/geront/gnq060

Engel, G. L. (1977). The need for a new medical model: A challenge for biomedicine. *Science, 196*(4286), 129–136. doi:10.1126/science.847460

Erikson, E. H. (1980). *Identity and the life cycle.* New York, NY: W. W. Norton & Company.

Erikson, E. H., & Erikson, J. M. (1997). *The life cycle completed.* New York, NY: Norton & Company.

Erikson, E. H., Erikson, J. M., & Kivinick, H. Q. (1986). *Vital involvement in old age: The experience of old age in our time.* New York, NY: Norton & Company.

Espinoza, R. (2012, September 27). Integrating LGBT older adults into the Older Americans Act. *The Huffington Post.* Retrieved from http://www.huffingtonpost.com/robert-espinoza/integrating-lgbt-older-ad_b_1917037.html

Fauci, A. S., Pantaleo, G., Stanley, S., & Weisman, D. (1996). Immunopathogenic mechanisms of HIV infection. *Annals of Internal Medicine, 124*(7), 654–663.

Fischl, M. A., Richman, D. D., Grieco, M. H., Gottlieb, M. S., Volberding, P. A., Laskin, O. L., ... King, D. (1987). The efficacy of azidothymidine (AZT) in the treatment of patients with AIDS and AIDS-related complex. *New England Journal of Medicine*, *317*(4), 185–191. doi:10.1056/NEJM198707233170401

Fox, M. J. (2009). *Always looking up: The adventures of an incurable optimist*. London, UK: Ebury Press.

France, D. (2013, February 1). Ed Koch and the AIDS crisis: His greatest failure. *New York Magazine*. Retrieved from http://nymag.com/daily/intelligencer/2013/02/koch-and-the-aids-crisis-his-greatest-failure.html

Gabriel, M. A. (1994). Group therapists and AIDS groups: An exploration of traumatic stress reactions. *GROUP*, *18*(3), 167–176. doi:10.1007/BF01456587

Gay Men's Health Crisis. (2010). *Growing older with the epidemic: HIV and aging*. New York, NY: Author.

Genke, J. (2004). Resistance and resilience. *Journal of Gay & Lesbian Social Services*, *17*(2), 81–95. doi:10.1300/J041v17n02_05

Gilligan, C. (1993). *In a different voice: Psychological theory and women's development*. Cambridge, MA: Harvard University Press.

Gilligan, C., Spencer, R., Weinberg, M. K., & Bertsch, T. (2003). On the listening guide: A voice-centered relational method. In P. M. Camic, J. E. Rhodes, & L. Yardley (Eds.), *Qualitative research in psychology: Expanding perspectives in methodology and design* (pp. 253–271). Washington, DC: American Psychological Association.

Gilmer, D. F., & Aldwin, C. M. (2003). *Health, illness, and optimal aging: Biological and psychosocial perspectives*. Thousand Oaks, CA: Sage Publications.

Goedert, J., Wallen, W., Mann, D., Strong, D., Neuland, C., Greene, M., ... Blattner, W. (1982). Amyl nitrite may alter T lymphocytes in homosexual men. *The Lancet*, *319*(8269), 412–416. doi:10.1016/S0140-6736(82)91617-8

Goldberg, N. G., & Gates, G. J. (2010). *Effects of lifting blood donation ban on men who have sex with men*. Los Angeles, CA: The Williams Institute.

Goldstein, R., & Massa, R. (1989, May 30). Compound Q: Hope and hype; the making of a new AIDS drug. *Village Voice*, pp. 29–34.

Goldstone, S. E. (2005). Diagnosis and treatment of HPV-Related squamous intraepithelial neoplasia in men who have sex with men. *The PRN Notebook*, *10*(4), 11–16.

Gottlieb, M. S., Schroff, R., Schanker, H. M., Weisman, J. D., Fan, P. T., Wolf, R. A., & Saxon, A. (1981). Pneumocystis carinii pneumonia and mucosal candidiasis in previously healthy homosexual men: Evidence of a new acquired cellular immunodeficiency. *New England Journal of Medicine*, *305*(24), 1425. doi:10.1056/NEJM198112103052401

Gran Fury, & Cohen, J. (2011). *Gran Fury: Read my lips*. New York, NY: 80wse Press, New York University.

Grant, R. M., Lama, J. R., Anderson, P. L., McMahan, V., Liu, A. Y., Vargas, L., ... Glidden, D. V. (2010). Preexposure chemoprophylaxis for HIV prevention in men who have sex with men. *New England Journal of Medicine*, *363*(27), 2587–2599. doi:10.1056/NEJMoa1011205

Gray, H., & Dressel, P. (1985). Alternative interpretations of aging among gay males. *The Gerontologist*, *25*(1), 83–87. doi:10.1093/geront/25.1.83

Grov, C., Golub, S. A., Parsons, J. T., Brennan, M., & Karpiak, S. E. (2010). Loneliness and HIV-related stigma explain depression among older HIV-positive adults. *AIDS Care, 22*(5), 630–639. doi:10.1080/09540120903280901

Halkitis, P. N. (1999). Redefining masculinity in the age of AIDS: Seropositive gay men and the "buff agenda." In P. Nardi (Ed.), *Gay masculinities* (pp. 130–151). Newbury Park, CA: Sage.

Halkitis, P. N. (2001). An exploration of perceptions of masculinity among gay men living with HIV. *Journal of Men's Studies, 9*(3), 413–429. doi:10.3149/jms.0903.413

Halkitis, P. N. (2005). Foreword. In M. Shernoff, *Without condoms: Unprotected sex, gay men & barebacking* (pp. viii–xviii). New York, NY: Routledge.

Halkitis, P. N. (2009). *Methamphetamine addiction: Biological foundations, psychological factors, and social consequences.* Washington, DC: APA Publications.

Halkitis, P. N. (2010a). Reframing HIV prevention for gay men in the United States. *American Psychologist, 65*(8), 752–763. doi:10.1037/0003-066X.65.8.752

Halkitis, P. N. (2010b, September 8). For HIV-positive men, 50 is the new 40 (and the new 60). *Chelsea Now, 4*(30), pp. 17–18.

Halkitis, P. N. (2011, November 30). Reflecting on the AIDS generation. *Chelsea Now, 4*(33), pp. 18–19.

Halkitis, P. N. (2012a). Discrimination and homophobia fuel the HIV epidemic in gay and bisexual men. *Psychology & AIDS Exchange, Spring,* 4–11.

Halkitis, P. N. (2012b). Obama, marriage equality, and the health of gay men. *American Journal of Public Health, 102*(9), 1628–1629. doi:10.2105/AJPH.2012.300940

Halkitis, P. N. (2013, March 8). HIV and the power of escape. *The Huffington Post.* Retrieved from http://www.huffingtonpost.com/perry-n-halkitis-phd-ms/the-aids-generation_b_2832058.html

Halkitis, P. N. & Marino, M. (2011, September 9). HIV researcher charts "terror sex" after 9/11. *Chelsea Now, 5*(4), p. 17.

Halkitis, P. N., Barton, S. C., & Blachman-Foshay, J. (2012, February, 22). Mythologies and misunderstandings of HIV-negative test results. *Chelsea Now, 4*(39), pp. 18–19.

Halkitis, P. N., & Blachman-Forshay, J. (2011, August 24). It's more than just HIV-duh it's HPV too. *Chelsea Now, 5*(3), p. 12.

Halkitis, P. N., & Cahill, S. (2011, May 27). Re-centering science in the fight against AIDS. *The Huffington Post.* Retrieved from http://www.huffingtonpost.com/perry-n-halkitis-phd-ms/recentering-science-in-th_b_868310.html

Halkitis, P. N., Gomez, C., & Wolitski, R. (Eds.). (2005). *HIV + sex: The psychological and interpersonal dynamics of HIV-seropositive gay and bisexual men's relationships.* Washington, DC: APA Publications.

Halkitis, P. N., Green, K., Remien, R. H., Stirratt M. J., Hoff, C., Wolitski, R. J., & Parsons, J. T. (2005). Seroconcordant sexual partnerings of HIV-seropositive gay and bisexual men. *AIDS, 19*(S1), S77–S86. doi:10.1097/01.aids.0000167354.09912.83

Halkitis, P. N., Green, K. A., & Wilton, L. (2004). Masculinity, body image, and sexual behavior in HIV-seropositive gay men: A two-phase behavioral investigation using the Internet. *International Journal of Men's Health, 3*(1), 27–42. doi:10.3149/jmh.0301.27

Halkitis, P. N., Kupprat, S. A., Hampton, M. E., Perez Figueroa, R., Kingdon, M., Eddy, J., & Ompad, D. C. (2013). Evidence for a syndemic in aging HIV-positive gay, bisexual, and other MSM: Implications for a holistic approach to prevention and healthcare. *Annals of Anthropological Practice, 36,* 363–384.

Halkitis, P. N., Moeller, R. W., Siconolfi, D. E., Storholm, E. D., Solomon, T. M., & Bub, K. L. (2012). Measurement model exploring a syndemic in emerging adult gay and bisexual men. *AIDS and Behavior, 17*(2), 662–673. doi:10.1007/s10461-012-0273-3

Halkitis, P. N., Pollock, J. A., Pappas, M. K., Dayton, A., Moeller, R. W., Siconolfi, D., & Solomon, T. (2011). Substance use in the MSM population of New York City in the era of HIV/AIDS. *Substance Use and Misuse, 46* (2–3), 274–273. doi:10.3109/1 0826084.2011.523265

Halkitis, P. N. & Siconolfi, D. E. (2010, November 17). A call for revised HIV testing strategy. *Chelsea Now, 4*(35), pp. 1, 5, 7.

Halkitis, P. N., & Wilton, L. (2005). The meanings of sex for HIV-positive gay and bisexual men: Emotion, physicality, and affirmations of self. In P. N. Halkitis, R. J. Wolitski, & C. Gomez (Eds.), *HIV + sex: The psychological and interpersonal dynamics of HIV-seropositive gay and bisexual men's relationships* (pp. 21–38). Washington, DC: APA Publications.

Halkitis, P. N., Wilton, L., Parsons, J. T., & Hoff, C. (2004). Correlates of sexual risk taking behaviour among HIV seropositive gay men in concordant primary partner relationships. *Psychology, Health, & Medicine, 9*(1), 99–113. doi:10.1080/1354850 0310001637788

Halkitis, P. N., Wolitski, R. W., & Millett, G. A. (2013). The HIV health disparity in gay, bisexual, and other MSM and a theory of syndemics. *American Psychologist, 68*(4), 261–273. doi: 10.1037/a0032746

Hazuda, D., & Kuo, L. (1997). Failure of AZT: A molecular perspective. *Nature Medicine, 3*(8), 836–837. doi:10.1038/nm0897-836

Healthcare Intelligence Network. (2006, September). Baby boomers' impact on healthcare: High demands, expectations met with a healthy dose of prevention. Retrieved from http://emmcareguide.com/media/babyboomersandhealthcare.pdf

Heckman, T. G., Kochman, A., & Sikkema, K. J. (2002). Depressive symptoms in older adults living with HIV disease: Application of the chronic illness quality of life model. *Journal of Mental Health and Aging, 8*(4), 267–279.

Herek, G. M., & Glunt, E. K. (1995). Identity and community among gay and bisexual men in the AIDS era: Preliminary findings from the Sacramento Men's Health Study. In G. M. Herek & B. Greene (Eds.), *AIDS, identity, and community: The HIV epidemic and lesbians and gay men* (pp. 55–84). Thousand Oaks, CA: Sage.

Herrman, H., Stewart, D. E., Diaz-Granados, N., Berger, E. L, Jackson, B., & Yuen, T. (2011). What is resilience? *Canadian Journal of Psychiatry, 56*(5), 258–265.

Hoff, C. C., Chakravarty, D., Beougher, S. C., Darbes, L. A., Dadasovich, R., & Neilands, T. B. (2009). Serostatus differences and agreements about sex with outside partners among gay male couples. *AIDS Education and Prevention, 21*(1), 25–38. doi:10.1521/aeap.2009.21.1.25

Horberg, M. A., Silverberg, M. J., Hurley, L. B., Towner, W. J., Klein, D. B., Bersoff-Matcha, S.,...Kovach, D. A. (2008). Effects of depression and selective serotonin reuptake inhibitor use on adherence to highly active antiretroviral therapy and on clinical outcomes in HIV infected patients. *Journal of Acquired Immune Deficiency Syndromes, 47*(3), 384–390. doi:10.1097/QAI.0b013e318160d53e

Hsiao, W., Anastasia, K., Hall, J., Goodman, M., Rimland, D., Ritenour, C. W. M., & Issa, M. M. (2009). Association between HIV status and positive prostate biopsy in a study of U.S. *Scientific World Journal, 9*(Annual 2009), 102–108. doi:10.1100/tsw.2009.20

Hunter, E. G. (2007). Beyond death: Inheriting the past and giving to the future, transmitting the legacy of one's self. *OMEGA: Journal of Death and Dying, 56*(4), 313–329. doi:10.2190/OM.56.4.a

Hunter, E. G., & Rowles, G. D. (2005). Leaving legacy: Toward a typology. *Journal of Aging Studies, 19*(3), 327–347. doi:10.1016/j.jaging.2004.08.002

Ickovics, J. R., Milan, S., Boland, R., Schoenbaum, E., Schuman, P., & Vlahov, D. (2006). Psychological resources protect heath: 5-year survival and immune function among HIV-infected women from four US cities. *AIDS, 20*(14), 1851–1860. doi:10.1097/01.aids.0000244204.95758.15

Ironson, G., Balbin, E., Stuetzle, R., Fletcher, M. A., O'Ceeirigh, C., Laurenceau, J. P.,... & Solomon, G. (2005). Dispositional optimism and the mechanism by which it predicts slower disease progression in HIV: Proactive behavior, avoidant coping, and depression. *International Journal of Behavioral Medicine, 12*(2), 86–97. doi:10.1207/s15327558ijbm1202_6

Ironson, G., & H'Sien, H. (2008). Do positive psychosocial factors predict disease progression in HIV-1? A review of the evidence. *Psychosomatic Medicine, 70*(5), 546–554. doi:10.1097/PSY.0b013e318177216c

Jobs, S. (2005, June 14). "You've got to find what you love: Job says. Stanford Report. Retrieved from http://news.stanford.edu/news/2005/june15/jobs-061505.html

Kapadia, F., Siconolfi, D. E., Barton, S., Olivieri, B., Lombardo, L., & Halkitis, P. N. (2013). Social network characteristics and sexual risk taking among a racially/ethnically diverse sample of young, urban men who have sex with men. *AIDS & Behavior, 17*(5), 1819–1821. doi:10.1007/s10461-013-0468-2

Kennedy, Q., Mather, M., & Carstensen, L. L. (2004). The role of motivation in the age-related positivity effect in autobiographical memory. *Psychological Science, 15*(3), 208–214. doi:10.1111/j.0956-7976.2004.01503011.x

King, S. D., & Orel, N. (2012). Midlife and older gay men living with HIV/AIDS: The influence of resiliency and psychosocial stress factors on heath needs. *Journal of Gay & Lesbian Social Services, 24*(4), 346–370. doi:10.1080/10538720.2012.721669

Kirk, J. B., & Goetz, M. B. (2009). Human immunodeficiency virus in an aging population, a complication of success. *Journal of the American Geriatrics Society, 57*(11), 2129–2138. doi:10.1111/j.1532-5415.2009.02494.x

Koetting, M. E. (1996). A group design for HIV-negative gay men. *Social Work, 41*(4), 407–415. doi:10.1093/sw/41.4.407

Kohli, R., Klein, R. S., Schoenbaum, E. E., Anastos, K., Minkoff, H., & Sacks, H. S. (2006). Aging and HIV infection. *Journal of Urban Health, 83*(1), 31–42. doi:10.1007/s11524-005-9005-6

Koopman, C., Classen, C., Cardeña, E., & Spiegel, D. (1995). When disaster strikes, acute stress disorder may follow. *Journal of Traumatic Stress, 8*(1), 29–46. doi:10.1007/BF02105405

Kramer, L. (2000). *The normal heart and the destiny of me: Two plays.* New York, NY: Grove Press.

Krieger, N. (2001). Theories for social epidemiology in the 21st century: An ecosocial perspective. *International Journal of Epidemiology*, *30*(4), 668–677. doi:10.1093/ije/30.4.668

Leland, J. (2013, June 2). 'People think it's over;' Spared death, aging people with HIV struggle to live. *The New York Times*. Retrieved from http://www.nytimes.com/2013/06/02/nyregion/spared-death-aging-people-with-hiv-struggle-to-live.html?pagewanted=all

Leserman, J. (2003). HIV disease progression: Depression, stress, and possible mechanisms. *Biological Psychiatry*, *54*(3), 295–306. doi:10.1016/S0006-3223(03)00323-8

Leserman, J., Jackson, E. D., Petitto, J. M., Golden, R. N., Silva, S. G., Perkins, D. O.,...Evans, D. L. (1999). Progression to AIDS: The effects of stress, depressive symptoms, and social support. *Psychosomatic Medicine*, *61*(3), 397–406.

Leserman, J., Petitto, J. M., Golden, R. N., Gaynes, B. N., Gu, H., Perkins, D. O.,...Evans, D. L. (2000). Impact of stressful life events, depression, social support, coping, and cortisol on progression to AIDS. *American Journal of Psychiatry*, *157*(8), 1221–1228. doi:10.1176/appi.ajp.157.8.1221

Leserman, J., Petitto, J. M., Gu, H., Gaynes, B. N., Barroso, J., Golden, R. N.,...Evans, D. L. (2002). Progression to AIDS, a clinical AIDS condition and mortality: Psychosocial and physiological predictors. *Psychological Medicine*, *32*(6), 1059–1073. doi:10.1017/S0033291702005949

Levine, J. (1986, September, 29). A ray of hope in the fight against AIDS. *Time Magazine*. Retrieved from http://www.time.com/time/magazine/article/0,9171,962389,00.html

Link, B. G., & Phelan, J. (1995). Social conditions as fundamental causes of disease. *Journal of Health and Social Behavior*, *35*(Extra Issue), 80–94. doi:10.2307/2626958

Louganis, G., & Marcus, E. (1995). *Breaking the surface*. New York, NY: Random House.

Luthar, S. (2006). Resilience in development: A synthesis of research across five decades. In D. Cicchetti & D. J. Cohen (Eds.), *Developmental psychopathology: Risk, disorder, and adaptation* (2nd ed., pp. 739–795). New York, NY: Wiley.

Machtinger, E. L., Wilson, T. C., Haberer, J. E., & Weiss, D. S. (2012). Psychological trauma and PTSD in HIV-positive women: A meta-analysis. *AIDS and Behavior*, *16*(9), 2091–2100. doi:10.1007/s10461-011-0127-4

Mancilla, M., & Troshinsky, L. (2003). *Love in the time of HIV: The gay man's guide to sex, dating, and relationships*. New York, NY: Guilford Publications.

Marshall, R. D., Spitzer, R., & Liebowitz, M. R. (1999). Review and critique of the new DSM-IV diagnosis of acute stress disorder. *American Journal of Psychiatry*, *156*(11), 1677–1685.

Massa, R. (1990, July 9). Unfit to print. *Village Voice*, *35*(19), pp. 24–26.

Massa, R. (1995). Specimen days. In M. Howe & M. Klein (Eds.), *In the company of my solitude: American writing from the AIDS pandemic* (pp. 168–175). New York, NY: Persea Books.

Masten, A. S., & Powell, J. L. (2003). A resiliency framework for research, policy and practice. In S. Luthar (Ed.), *Resiliency and vulnerability: Adaptation in the context of childhood adversity* (pp. 1–29). Cambridge, UK: Cambridge University Press.

Mather, M., & Johnson, M. K. (2000). Choice-supportive source monitoring: Do our decisions seem better to us as we age? *Psychology and Aging*, *15*(4), 596–606. doi:10.1037/0882-7974.15.4.596

McAdams, D. P. (1993). *The stories we live by: Personal myths and making of the self.* New York, NY: William Morrow & Co.

McNeil, D. G. (2012, July 3). Rapid H.I.V. home test wins federal approval. *The New York Times.* Retrieved from http://www.nytimes.com/2012/07/04/health/oraquick-at-home-hiv-test-wins-fda-approval.html

Medapalli, R. K., Parikh, C. R., Gordon, K., Brown, S. T., Butt, A. A., Gibert, C. L.,...Wyatt, C. M. (2012). Comorbid diabetes and the risk of progressive chronic kidney disease in HIV-infected adults: Data from the Veterans Aging Cohort Study. *Journal of Acquired Immune Deficiency Syndromes, 60*(4), 393–399. doi:10.1097/QAI.0b013e31825b70d9

Milam, J. E., Richardson, J. L., Marks, G., Kemper, C. A., & McCutchan, A. J. (2004). The roles of dispositional optimism and pessimism in HIV disease progression. *Psychology & Health, 19*(2), 167–181.

Military HIV Research Program. (2012). *U.S. military HIV research program.* Retrieved from http://www.hivresearch.org/about.php?AboutusID=6

Miller, A. (1997). *The drama of the gifted child: The search for the true self.* New York, NY: Basic Books.

Mills, E. J., Bärnighausen, T., & Negin, J. (2012). HIV and aging--preparing for the challenges ahead. *New England Journal of Medicine, 366*(14), 1270–1273. doi:10.1056/NEJMp1113643

Monette, P. (1988). *Borrowed time: An AIDS memoir.* San Diego, CA: Harcourt Brace Javanovich.

Moremen, R. D. (2005). What is the meaning of life? Women's spirituality at the end of the lifespan. *OMEGA: Journal of Death and Dying, 50*(4), 309–330. doi:10.2190/X36M-F7XQ-PENB-RFBF

Murray, J., & Adam, B. D. (2001). Aging, sexuality, and HIV issues among older gay men. *Canadian Journal of Human Sexuality, 10*(3/4), 75–90.

Myers, J. D. (2009). Growing old with HIV: The AIDS epidemic and an aging population. *Journal of the American Academy of Physician Assistants, 22*(1), 20–24.

Nakagawa, F., Lodwock, R. K. Smith, C. J., Smith, R., Cambiano, V., Lundgren, J. D.,...& Philips, A. N. (2012). Projected life expectancy of people with HIV according to timing of diagnosis. *AIDS, 26*(3), 335–343. doi:10.1097/QAD.0b013e32834dcec9

O'Cleirigh, C., Ironson, G., Antoni, M., Fletcher, M. A., McGuffey, E. B.,...& Solomon, G. (2003). Emotional expression and depth processing of trauma and their relation to long-term survival in patients with HIV/AIDS. *Journal of Psychosomatic Research, 54*(3), 225–235. doi:10.1016/S0022-3999(02)00524-X

O'Cleirigh, C., Ironson, G., Fletcher, M. A., & Schneiderman, N. (2008).Written emotional disclosure and processing of trauma are associated with protected health status and immunity in people living with HIV/AIDS. *British Journal of Health Psychology, 13*(1), 81–84. doi:10.1348/135910707X250884

Odets, W. (1995). *In the shadow of the epidemic: Being HIV-negative in the age of AIDS.* Durham, NC: Duke University Press Books.

Omoto, A. M., & Crain, A. L. (1995). AIDS volunteerism: Lesbian and gay community-based responses to HIV. In G. M. Herek & B. Greene (Eds.), *AIDS, identity, and community: The HIV epidemic and lesbians and gay men* (pp. 187–209). Thousand Oaks, CA: Sage.

Osmond, D. H. (2008). Epidemiology of disease progression in HIV. *HIV Insite Knowledge Base Chapter*. Retrieved from http://hivinsite.ucsf.edu/InSite?page=kb-03-01-04

Oswald, G. A., Theodossi, A., Gazzard, B. G., Byrom, N. A., & Fisher-Hoch, S. P. (1982). Attempted immune stimulation in the "gay compromise syndrome". *British Medical Journal (Clinical Research Ed.)*, *285*(6348), 1082. doi:10.1136/bmj.285.6348.1082

Owen, G., & Catalan, J. (2012). "We never expected this to happen": Narratives of ageing with HIV among gay men living in London, UK. *Culture, Health and Sexuality*, *14*(1), 59–72. doi:10.1080/13691058.2011.621449

Palefsky, J. E. (2005). Screening and treatment of anal intraepithelial neoplasia to prevent anal cancer: Where do we stand? *The PRN Notebook*, *10*(4), 17–18.

Palella Jr., F. J., Baker, R. K., Moorman, A. C., Chmiel, J. S., Wood, K. C., Brooks, J. T., & Holmberg, S. D. (2006). Mortality in the highly active antiretroviral therapy era: Changing causes of death and disease in the HIV outpatient study. *Journal of Acquired Immune Deficiency Syndrome*, *43*(1), 27–34. doi:10.1097/01.qai.0000233310.90484.16

Palella Jr., F. J., Delaney, K. M., Moorman, A. C., Loveless, M. O., Fuhrer, J., Satten, G. A., ... & Holmberg, S. D. (1998). Declining morbidity and mortality among patients with advanced human immunodeficiency virus infection. *New England Journal of Medicine*, *338*(13), 853–860. doi:10.1056/NEJM199803263381301

Parsons, J. T., Vicioso, K., Punzalan, J. C., Halkitis, P. N., Kutnick, A., & Velasquez, M. M. (2004). The impact of alcohol use on the sexual scripts of HIV-positive men who have sex with men. *Journal of Sex Research*, *41*(2), 160–172. doi:10.1080/00224490409552224

Paterson, D. L., Swindells, S., Mohr, J., Brester, M., Vergis, E. N., Squier, C., ... Singh, N. (2000). Adherence to protease inhibitor therapy and outcomes in patients with HIV infection. *Annals of Internal Medicine*, *133*(1), 21–30.

Pear, R. (1985, March 3). AIDS blood test to be available in 2 to 6 weeks. *The New York Times*. Retrieved from http://www.nytimes.com/1985/03/03/us/aids-blood-test-to-be-available-in-2-to-6-weeks.html

Pennebaker, J. W., Kiecolt-Glaser, J. K., & Glaser, R. (1988). Disclosure of traumas and immune function: Health implications for psychotherapy. *Journal of Consulting and Clinical Psychology*, *56*(2), 239–245. doi:10.1037/0022-006X.56.2.239

Perez Figueroa, R., & Halkitis, P. N. (2012, June 15). Anal health: Getting to the bottom of the matter. *Chelsea Now, 4*(47), pp. 19–20.

Platzer, C., Döcke, W. D., Volk, H. D., & Prösch, S. (2000). Catecholamines trigger IL-10 release in acute systemic stress reaction by direct stimulation of its promoter/enhancer activity in monocytic cells. *Journal of Neuroimmunology*, *105*(1), 31–38. doi:10.1016/S0165-5728(00)00205-8

Popovic, M., Sarngadharan, M. G., Read, E., & Gallo, R. C. (1984). Detection, isolation, and continuous production of cytopathic retroviruses (HTLV-III) from patients with AIDS and pre-AIDS. *Science, 224*(4648), 497–500. doi:10.1126/science.6200935

Poundstone, K. E., Strathdee, S. A., & Celentano, D. D. (2004). The social epidemiology of human immunodeficiency virus/acquired immune deficiency syndrome. *Epidemiological Reviews*, *26*(1), 22–35. doi:10.1093/epirev/mxh005

Public Broadcasting Service. (2012). *Margaret Mitchell: American rebel; interview with Margaret Mitchell from 1936; The Atlanta Journal*. Retrieved from http://www.pbs.org/wnet/americanmasters/episodes/margaret-mitchell-american-rebel/interview-with-margaret-mitchell-from-1936/2011/

Purcell, D. W., Ibanez, G. E., & Schwatz, D. J. (2005). Under the influence: Alcohol and drug use and sexual behavior among HIV-positive gay and bisexual men. In P. N. Halkitis, R. J. Wolitski, & C. Gomez (Eds.), *HIV + sex: The psychological and interpersonal dynamics of HIV-seropositive gay and bisexual men's relationships* (pp. 163–182). Washington, DC: APA Publications.

Rapp, C. (1998). *The strengths model: Case management with people suffering from severe and persistent mental illness.* New York, NY: Oxford University Press.

Rayburn, C. A. (2008). Clinical and pastoral issue and challenges in working with the dying and their families. *Adultspan Journal, 7*(2), 94–108. doi:10.1002/j.2161-0029.2008. tb00049.x

Reed, G. M., Kemeny, M. E., Taylor, S. E., Wang, H. Y. J., & Visscher, B. R. (1994). Realistic acceptance as a predictor of decreased survival time in gay men with AIDS. *Health Psychology, 13*(4), 299–307. doi:10.1037/0278-6133.13.4.299

Reeves, P. M., Merriam, S. B., & Courtenay, B. C. (1999). Adaptation to HIV infection: The development of coping strategies over time. *Qualitative Health Research, 9*(3), 344–361. doi:10.1177/104973299129121901

Reinhberg, S. (2012, November 29). New HIV infections highest among urban gay, bisexual men: CDC. *U.S. News and World Report.* Retrieved from http://health. usnews.com/health-news/news/articles/2012/11/29/new-hiv-infections-highest-among-urban-gay-bisexual-men-cdc

Remien, R. H., & Rabkin, J. G. (1995). Long-term survival with AIDS and the role of community. In G. M. Herek & B. Greene (Eds.), *AIDS, identity, and community: The HIV epidemic and lesbians and gay men* (pp. 169–186). Thousand Oaks, CA: Sage.

Remien, R. H., Wagner, G., Dolezal, C., & Carballo-Dieguez, A. (2002). Factors associated with HIV sexual risk behavior in male couples of mixed HIV status. *Journal of Psychology and Human Sexuality, 13*(3), 31–48. doi:10.1300/J056v13n02_03

Resnick, M. D. (2000). Protective factors, resiliency, and healthy youth development. *Adolescent Medicine: State of the Art Reviews, 11*(1), 157–164.

Richman, D. D., Fischl, M. A., Grieco, M. H., Gottlieb, M. S., Volberding, P. A., Laskin, O. L.,…Nusinoff-Lehrman, S. (1987). The toxicity of azidothymidine (AZT) in the treatment of patients with AIDS and AIDS-related complex. *New England Journal of Medicine, 317*(4), 192–197. doi:10.1056/NEJM198707233170402

Rivero, J., Fraga, M., Cancio, I., Cuervo, J., & Lopez-Saura, P. (1997). Long term treatment with recombinant interferon alpha-2b prolongs survival of asymptomatic HIV-infected individuals. *Biotherapy, 10*(2), 107–113. doi:10.1007/BF02678537

Roberts, S. (2012, September 2). A history of New York in 50 objects. *The New York Times.* Retrieved from http://query.nytimes.com/gst/fullpage.html?res=9D00E2D91 03CF931A3575AC0A9649D8B63&ref=americanmuseumofnaturalhistory

Rodgers, R., & Hammerstein, O. (1942). *Oklahoma.* Retrieved from http://www.system-eyescomputerstore.com/scripts/Oklahoma/index.html

Roosa, M. W. (2000). Some thoughts about resilience versus positive development, main effects versus interactions, and the value of resilience. *Child Development, 71*(3), 567–569. doi:10.1111/1467-8624.00166

Rosenfeld, D., Bartlam, B., & Smith, R. D. (2012). Out of the closet and into the trenches: Gay male baby boomers, aging, and HIV/AIDS. *The Gerontologist, 52*(2), 255–264. doi:10.1093/geront/gnr138

Rotello, G. (1997). *Sexual ecology: AIDS and the destiny of gay men.* New York, NY: Dutton.

Russo, V. (1987). *The celluloid closet: Homosexuality in the movies* (Rev. ed.). New York, NY: Harper & Row.

Rutter, M. (1987). Psychosocial resilience and protective mechanisms. *American Journal of Orthopsychiatry, 57*(3), 316–331. doi:10.1111/j.1939-0025.1987.tb03541.x

Ryan, C., Russell, S. T., Huebner, D., Diaz, R., & Sanchez, J. (2010). Family acceptance in adolescence and the health of LGBT young adults. *Journal of Child and Adolescent Psychiatric Nursing, 23*(4), 205–213. doi:10.1111/j.1744-6171.2010.00246.x

Sadler-Gerhardt, C. J., & Hollenbach, J. G. (2011). Legacy work: Helping clients with life-threatening illness to preserve memories, beliefs, and values for loved ones. *VISTAS Online—American Counseling Association.* Retrieved from http://www.counseling.org/resources/library/vistas/2011-V-Online/Article_95.pdf

SAGE, & MAP. (2010, March). Improving the lives of LGBT older adults. Retrieved from http://www.lgbtmap.org/file/improving-the-lives-of-lgbt-older-adults.pdf

Salyer, D. (1999, June). The reinfection debate. *The Body.* Retrieved from http://www.thebody.com/content/art32373.html

Schonnesson, L. N. (2002). Psychological and existential issues and quality of life in people living with HIV infection. *AIDS Care, 14*(3), 399–404. doi:10.1080/09540120220123784

Shernoff, M. (2005). Without condoms: Unprotected sex, gay men & barebacking. New York, NY: Routledge.

Shilts, R. (1987). *And the band played on: People, politics, and the AIDS epidemic.* New York, NY: St. Martins.

Siegel, K., & Lekas, H-M. (2002). AIDS as chronic illness: Psychosocial implications. *AIDS, 16*(suppl 4): S69–S76. doi:10.1097/00002030-200216004-00010

Siegel, K., Raveis, V., & Karus, D. (1998). Perceived advantages and disadvantages of age among older HIV-infected adults. *Research on Aging, 20*(6), 686–711. doi:10.1177/0164027598206004

Slavin, S., Elliott, J., Fairley, C., French, M., Hoy, J., Law, M., & Lewin, S. (2011). HIV and aging: An overview of an emerging issue. *Sexual Health, 8*(4), 449–451. doi:10.1071/SH11110

Solano, L., Costa, M., Slavati, S., Coda, R., Aiuti, F., Mezzaroma, I., & Bertini, M. (1993). Psychosocial factors and clinical evolution of HIV-infection: A longitudinal study. *Journal of Psychosomatic Research, 37*(1), 39–51.

Sontag, S. (1977). *Illness as metaphor.* New York, NY: Vintage Books.

Stall, R., Friedman, M., & Catania, J. A. (2008). Interacting epidemics and gay men's health: A theory of syndemic production among urban gay men. In R. J. Wolitski, R. Stall, & R. O. Valdiserri (Eds.), *Unequal opportunity: Health disparities affecting gay and bisexual men in the United States* (pp. 251–274). Oxford, UK: Oxford University Press. Sullivan, A. (1999). Love undetectable: notes on friendship, sex, and survival. New York, NY: Vintage.

Sullivan, A. (1999). Love undetectable: notes on friendship, sex, and survival. New York, NY: Vintage.

Stephenson, R., Sullivan, P. S., Salazar, L. F., Gratzer, B., Allen, S., & Seelbach, E. (2011). Attitudes towards couples-based HIV testing among MSM in three US cities. *AIDS and Behavior, 15*(1), 80–87. doi:10.1007/s10461-011-9893-2

Sullivan, P. S., Salazar, L., Buchbinder, S., & Sanchez, T. H. (2009). Estimating the proportion of HIV transmissions from main sex partners among men who have sex with men in five US cities. *AIDS, 23*(9), 1153–1162. doi:10.1097/QAD.0b013e32832baa34

Szmuness W. (2005). Large-scale efficacy trials of hepatitis B vaccines in the USA: Baseline data and protocols. *Journal of Medical Virology, 4*(4), 327–340.

Theorell, T., Blomjvist, V., Jonsson, H., Schulman, S., Berntorp, E., & Stigendal, L. (1995). Social support and the development of immune function in human immunodeficiency virus infection. *Psychosomatic Medicine, 57*(1), 32–36.

Tien, P. C., Choi, A. I., Zolopa, A. R., Benson, C., Tracy, R., Scherzer, R.,... & Grunfedl, C. (2010). Inflammation and mortality in HIV-infected adults: Analysis of the FRAM study cohort. *Journal of Acquired Immune Deficiency Syndrome, 55*(3), 316–322.

Trautwein, M. (2011, June 5). The death sentence that defined my life. *The New York Times.* Retrieved from http://www.nytimes.com/2011/06/05/opinion/05trautwein.html?pagewanted=all&_r=0

Valente, S. M. (2003). Depression and HIV. *Journal of the Association of Nurses in AIDS Care, 14*(2), 41–51. doi:10.1177/1055329002250993

Vallet-Pichard, A., Mallet, V., & Pol, S. (2012). Nonalcoholic fatty liver disease and HIV infection. *Seminars in Liver Disease, 32*(2), 158–166. doi:10.1055/s-0032-1316471

Vance, D. E. & Woodley, R. A. (2005). Strengths and distress in adults who are aging with HIV: a pilot study. *Psychological Reports, 96*(2), 383–386. doi:10.2466/pr0.96.2.383-386

Van Wagenen, A., Driskell, J., & Bradford, J. (2013). "I'm still raring to go": Successful aging among lesbian, gay, bisexual, and transgender adults. *Journal of Aging Studies, 27*(1), 1–14.

Wagnild, G. (2003). Resilience and successful aging: Comparison among low and high income older adults. *Journal of Gerontological Nursing, 29*(12), 42–49.

Wagnild, G. (2009). A review of the resilience scale. *Journal of Nursing Measurement, 17*(2), 105–113.

Walker A. K. (2011, October 2). Once resigned to die, the afflicted get older. *The Miami Herald*, p. 5A.

Weeks, B. S., & Alcamo, I. E. (2010). *AIDS: The biological basis.* Boston, MA: Jones and Bartlett.

Weitz, R. (1989). Uncertainty in the lives of persons with AIDS. *Journal of Health and Social Behavior, 30*(3), 270–281.

West, T. M. (1994). Psychological issues in hospice music therapy. *Music Therapy Perspectives, 12*(2), 117–124.

Whitehead, M., & Diderichsen, F. (2001). Social capital and health: Tip-toeing through the minefield of evidence. *The Lancet, 358*(9277), 165–166.

White House Office of National AIDS Policy. (2010, July). *The national HIV/AIDS strategy.* Washington, DC: Author.

Woods, S. P., Moore, D. J., Weber, E., & Grant, I. (2009). Cognitive neuropsychology of HIV-associated neurocognitive disorders. *Neuropsychology Review, 19*(2), 152–168.

World Health Organization (2011, November 30). *Global HIV/AIDS response: Epidemic update and health sector progress towards universal access. Progress*

Report 2011. Retrieved from http://www.who.int/hiv/pub/progress_report2011/en/index.html

Yabrov, A. (2000). It is hazardous to treat HIV patients with interferon-a. *Medical Hypotheses, 54*(1), 131–136.

Zautra, A. J., Hall, J. S., & Murray, K. E. (2010). Resilience: A new definition of health for people and communities. In J. W. Reich, A. J. Zautra, & J. S. Hall (Eds.), *Handbook of adult resilience* (pp. 3–29). New York, NY: Guilford Press.

Zogg, J. B., Woods, S. P., Sauceda, J. A., Wiebe, J. S., & Simoni, J. M. (2012). The role of prospective memory in medication adherence: a review of an emerging literature. *Journal of Behavioral Medicine, 35*(1), 47–62.

INDEX

"f" indicates material in footnotes and "t" indicates material in tables.

Bayer, Ronald, 86

Bennet, Michael (Senator), 188

Bennett, Michael, 84, 177

Bergeron, Bob, 188

Bernstein, Jacob, 192

Biological legacy, 144

Biomedical model, 197–198, 205

Biopsychosocial framework, 97–100, 189, 197–198, 201–202, 205

Bobby
childhood of, 30–32, 208
on computer pornography, 133
description of, 30–32
Eriksonian perspective of, 142–143
on HIV-prevention outreach, 182
on legacy, 150
on new generation of HIV-positive men, 180, 210, 213
on positive test, 62, 72–73, 80
resilience of, 203, 205
substance use by, 81, 109, 133, 134, 198–199
suicide attempt by, 133
survival strategies of, 126, 133
on survivor's guilt, 153
on wedding, 141, 203

Body Positive, 100, 118, 178

Body Positive, The, 118

Borrowed Time (Monette), 59

Broadway Cares, 44

"Bug chasing," 151

Bullying, 32–33, 184, 208

Bush, George W., 3

Butyl nitrate, 2

Byrne, Angela, 216–217

Cahill, Sean, 7, 184, 187

Callen, Michael, 6, 21, 76, 81, 103, 135

Cancer, 3, 4, 167, 170. See also specific types

Cardiovascular disease, 167

Catalan, Jose, 140, 152, 157

CD4/T-cell counts, 82

Center for Health, Identity, Behavior, and Prevention Studies (CHIBPS)
anal cancer articles by, 169–170
HIV/AIDS research by, xiv, 8–10
Project Gold. See Project Gold

Centers for Disease Control and Prevention (CDC)
on AIDS, 82
case guidelines from, 82
on HIV, 82
on holistic approaches, 115
on middle-age HIV-positive men, 167
mortality data from, 56, 78
MSM criterion of, 2, 17, 167
prevalence data from, 2, 190–191

Central Park (Rambles), 51

Cerebrovascular disease, 167

Cervical cancer, 170

Cherry Grove on Fire Island, 175

CHIBPS. See Center for Health, Identity, Behavior, and Prevention Studies

Chinese cucumber, 5, 102

Chlamydia, 9

Cholesterol, 168

Christopher
childhood of, 39
on dating, 186
on death and dying, 159, 165
description of, 37, 38–41
emotional health of, 112–114
on family, 185, 206
on legacy, 146
on life after HIV diagnosis, 96, 98–100
on new generation of HIV-positive men, 183, 186, 213
peers, connections to, 163
on positive test, 41, 62, 66–67, 75
resilience of, 194–195, 199, 206–207

Egrifta, 212

ELISA, 57

Emotional abuse, 161, 204

Enzyme-linked immunosorbent assay (ELISA), 57

Epigenetic approach, 95–97

Epivir. *See* 3TC

Erikson, Erik H., 95–97, 141–143, 146–147

Ethnicity, 2, 9–10

Executive function, 168

Existential questions, 96

"Expected positives," 72–75

Faith healers, 103, 135

Falwell, Jerry, 3

Farmer, Paul, 192

FDA, 64

"Fighter," 136

Fire Island Pines Property Owners Association Charitable Foundation, 54–55

Focus group meeting, 23–24

Food and Drug Administration (FDA), 64

Fox, Michael J., 213–214

France, David
  on Cox, ix–xi
  documentary. *See How to Survive a Plague*
  on Koch, 192
  resilience of, 203

Gallo, Robert, 57

Gay civil rights movement, 3–5, 12, 184, 207

Gay men
  appearance expectations of, 172–174
  behavioral research on, 11–12
  dating, 186
  media portrayals of, 4, 12, 180
  mental health of, 188
  population statistics on, 2, 179
  resilience model for, 12
  victimization of, 188
  in youth-obsessed culture, 174–176

Gay Men's Health Crisis (GMHC)
  alternative treatments offered at, 103
  death, dying, and, 80, 84
  group therapy at, 111
  HIV prevention approaches of, 184
  Morning Party, 54
  The Normal Heart on, 36
  outreach by, 182
  social networking at, 37
  social support from, 77, 116, 118, 120

"Gay Plague, The" (Alert Citizens of Texas), 3

Gay Pride, 116

Gay publications, 177

Gay-related immune deficiency (GRID), 2, 52, 73, 80, 81, 94

Geffen, David, 84

Generativity, 141–142, 146, 148, 189

Genke, John, 208, 209

Gianni
  childhood of, 29–30, 42, 209
  on death and dying, 88–89
  description of, 29–30
  on life after HIV diagnosis, 30, 101
  on medications, 168
  on middle-age, 138, 166–167
  on new generation of gay men, 181
  on physical health, 169
  on positive test, 30, 63, 69–70, 72, 108, 200
  resilience of, 200, 205, 209
  on September 11 terrorist attacks, 133
  social strategies of, 172
  survival strategies of, 122, 136
  young adult years of, 43–44

Lipodystrophy, 52, 55, 171–172

Listening Guide Method of Psychological Inquiry (Gilligan et al.), 11

Liver, 65, 167

London, 140, 216–217

Long Island Association for AIDS Care, 99

Long-term survivors
attitude of, 129
Barroso on, 81
Callen on, 6, 21, 81
Davies on, 81–82
guilt of, 152
Halkitis on, 7
new generation of gay men and, 210
in Project Gold, 10

Longtime Companion, 74, 76, 82

Louganis, Greg, 4, 58, 78

Love Heals, 32

Love in the Time of HIV (Mancilla & Troshinsky), 106

Love Undetectable (Sullivan), 173

Lungs, 167

Lymphadenopathy-associated virus (LAV), 57

Lymphoma, 5, 57, 170

MACS, 60

Managnier, Luc, 57

MAP, 188

Massa, Robert
on AZT, 5
complementary therapy use by, 5, 102–103
death of, 5, 6, 86, 91
editing *The Body Positive*, 118
foreword for *Without Condoms* on, 177
legacy of, 147
PML and, 92
survivor's guilt and, 155
TAG and, 192

Material legacy, 144

Measles, 41

Medius Working Group, 189

Meningitis, 212

"Men who have sex with men" (MSM), 2, 17, 167

Mermin, Jonathan, 191

Methamphetamines, x

MHRP, 67

Miami Herald, 7

Middle age
appearance expectations and, 171–174
CDC on men with HIV in, 167
Eriksonian perspective on, 97, 141–143
legacy framework for, 144–150
life course perspective on, 157
painful memories of loss in, 140–141, 144
past choices in context of, 143–144, 164–165
physical health and, 166–171
reflections on achieving, 138–140, 158–164
resilience model for, 143
sense- and meaning-making in, 156–157, 165–166, 216–217
survivor's guilt in, 151–155
in youth-obsessed culture, 175–176

Military HIV Research Program (MHRP), 67

Milk, Harvey, 4, 53

Mitchell, Margaret, 190

Monette, Paul, 59

Mood disorders, 168

Moral Majority Report, 3

Mormonism, 26

Morning Party, 54

Movement Advancement Project (MAP), 188

MSM, 2, 17, 167